THE MATURE
SOCIETY

THE MATURE SOCIETY

Dennis Gabor

PRAEGER PUBLISHERS
New York • Washington

301
Gllm
81796
Jan. 1973

BOOKS THAT MATTER

Published in the United States of America in 1972
by Praeger Publishers, Inc.
111 Fourth Avenue, New York, N.Y. 10003

© 1972 in London, England, by Dennis Gabor

Library of Congress Catalog Card Number: 72-75690

Printed in the United States of America

ACKNOWLEDGMENTS

I am grateful to Professor Jay W. Forrester, of the Massachusetts Institute of Technology, for having let me read the manuscript of his book *World Dynamics* before publication, and for permission to reproduce three of his illustrations.

I cannot give sufficient thanks to my brother André Gabor for his liberal assistance with ideas, data and criticism, and to my wife Marjorie for her great and constant love.

DENNIS GABOR
26 April 1971

CONTENTS

FOREWORD

This book is a sequel to my *Inventing the Future*, published in 1963. In that book I sketched the history and the present trends of our unique civilization, which is based materially on the solid foundation of scientific technology and spiritually on almost nothing. 'Till now man has been up against Nature; from now on he will be up against his own nature.' The age-old enemy, poverty, is defeated in one-quarter of the world, almost all the ailments which used to kill one-half of the people in childhood are eliminated; there is no enemy left but man. We have every right to be proud when we look back, none at all for pride when looking forward. The tragic situation has arisen that the very talents which have made the naked ape the master of the Earth are now turning against him; his fighting temper, his restless quest for novelty, his craving for excitement and adventure, even his virtues – such as the love and care for his progeny, and his social instincts which make him willing to sacrifice himself for his tribe or for his nation.

Science in combination with nationalism has created a situation in which a total war could wipe out all civilization. Science in combination with love for progeny has created overpopulation, the explosive multiplication of mankind. Science in combination with the old economic virtues has created techniques which can virtually eliminate work, the most harmless occupation of man, and have brought us face to face with an Age of Leisure, for which we are psychologically unprepared.

In the eight years since I wrote my first book, anxious preoccupation with the future has become very intense among the creative minorities of all industrial countries. More and more thinking people have realized that our free industrial civilization, which, with all its faults, is far superior to most systems of the past, not only in material success but also in humanity, is not likely to survive another generation without fundamental institutional changes. They are anxious lest social inertia might prevent gradual adaptation, until a critical point is reached at which the fear of a collapse by inner or outer pressure might drive the free countries into some sort of totalitarianism.

These forebodings are not unjustified. The atmosphere of fear arises from two sources. One is that in the last seven years Soviet policy has taken a turn towards a priority of armaments and power politics, as demonstrated in 1968 by the military occupation of Czechoslovakia, and by the spread of Soviet influence in the Middle East. The other source of fear is the moral erosion in the non-communist countries, which manifests itself in the rebellion of the university youth. Without attributing too much importance to the cult of violence nurtured by the extremist wing, the fact remains that a more than negligible fraction of our young people do not consider the consumer society interesting enough to live for. Added to this, increasing difficulties are experienced in the management of the economic system.

Until the last few years the highly industrialized countries had grown steadily in affluence. This was due not so much to Adam Smith's 'invisible hand' (which, as if by a miracle, coordinates private and public interests) as to the very visible hand of technology, which all the time kept creating new wealth for all. There would have been no need to worry if this growth had been *organic*, like the development of a living organism towards maturity, but much of it was just quantitative, not evolutionary. *Growth addiction* has become the universal creed of our world. This creed knows no ideological frontier: the American corporation president and his opposite number in the USSR both had to have a rising chart behind their desks – more production every year, be it in missiles, in motor cars or in baby food. The last appears to be the most harmless, but in the long run we can just as little afford overpopulation as we can afford war.

In this last quarter-century of steadily increasing affluence few people dared to face the obvious fact that exponential growth cannot be continued indefinitely. *Growth had become synonymous with hope*, and man cannot live without hope. Under the day-to-day pressure of business even highly intelligent people refused to think of the long term, and if they thought about it at all, they unconsciously repeated St Augustine's prayer: 'Lord, make me good, but not yet!' Let exponential growth continue in my time!

It now appears that a crisis is upon us, long before most people expected it. First in Britain, then a little later in the United States, production growth slowed down and even came to a temporary stop, while prices went up steadily, in spite of growing unemployment. The present crisis will certainly pass away, production will rise again through new technological improvements, though their introduction will be slowed down by the restriction on capital investments which was necessary to prevent runaway inflation. But the causes will remain with us, and I believe that they will be felt again in new crises. It is my belief that the present crisis is already a crisis of *saturation*, foreseen by J. M. Keynes forty years ago, but fervently disbelieved by most economists in the long period of year-to-year growth. In the UK and in the USA it manifests itself clearly in the unwillingness of the workers to work more in order to consume more.

Does this mean that the Age of Leisure is already partly with us, and that a new, reasonable equilibrium is announcing itself? I would say that the end of the dynamically growing consumer society is coming into sight, but the transition period will be neither stable nor happy. The vacant minds created by the consumer society will miss the Gospel of Work. For a while they might enjoy the visible protest which manifests itself in strikes, and in the more important silent protest of voluntary absenteeism, which is already strong in Britain and in the States. It is important in a free society to leave legitimate outlets for protest. It is greatly preferable to the practice in the totalitarian states where strikes are illegal and uncertified illness is punishable. But protest, though it is an important abstraction, is hardly an adequate foundation for a new, higher civilization.

In this book I have tried to sketch out a *Mature Society*; a peaceful world on a high level of material civilization, which has given up growth in numbers and in material consumption but not growth in the quality of life, and one which is compatible with the nature of *homo sapiens*. This last condition is a very hard one. The conquest of Nature by rational man, who has created science and technology, has brought us face to face with the basic irrationality of man. This I consider as an objective danger, as objective as floods, epidemics and bad harvests were yesterday. (And still are, in half of the world.) Irrational Man craves security, he will fight for it, but he despises it as soon as it is won. In the front line the soldier just wants to live; a little behind it he gets hungry, further behind he feels the stirrings of sex, and so on, until in full security he gets bored with it all and wants to fight something.

Man can be wonderful in adversity; he is liable to become a poor, aimless creature in security and affluence. Without his indomitable fighting spirit civilization would never have developed, nor would history be such a sad tale of violence and inhumanity. Whatever feelings one may have for the heroic struggles of the past, at the present stage of technological civilization the urge towards power over other men has become an unmitigated danger. Let the power which bio-engineering will give to the rulers fall into the wrong hands, and we shall have Orwellian hell.

Shall we be able to overcome the multitude of obstacles in a world organized for power and ruled by fear; can we effect what amounts almost to a mutation in the nature of men? I do not know the answer, I know only that we must not give up trying. It is the duty of every thinking man and woman to do their best to bring about a gradual turn from explosive, uncontrolled growth into organic development towards a mature society. I appeal to the inventive spirit of a whole generation. I wish they could be made to see that the invention of the future is not only infinitely more important, but also intellectually more rewarding than the 'conquest' of the planetary system.

As in my previous book, I have abstained from painting a Utopia, though I could not avoid sketching in a few of its features. We must think farther ahead than the politicians, who are worried to distraction by day-to-day emergencies, but we must not think too far ahead, or we come up against the unanswerable question of the 'ultimate aim of humanity'. But we can put up *signposts*: 'this way towards stability, that way into chaos.' Even if we cannot trace out the precise path towards a stable future, there is no excuse for going the opposite way, as is now only too often the case. Let us avoid the greatest dangers, while leaving as much freedom as possible for those who come after us, or else there will be no freedom in an overcrowded world, full of tensions. The rulers of the nations, at the end of their tether, might be tempted towards 'the last refuge of a scoundrel': the Police State.

This book consists roughly of two halves. In the first nine chapters I collect my data, in the other eleven I try to make constructive suggestions. I do not claim originality for all of them. In my scientific work I was accustomed to giving credit scrupulously to the originators of ideas; I regret that this is not possible in social science. I have relegated most of the statistical and technical material to the Notes, but I could not avoid quantitative discussions in some of the chapters (especially 9, 10 and 18), much as I regret that these may be somewhat difficult for readers with a literary-historical background to follow.

I have said very little about the technological novelties which may be expected in the near future, because these I have treated in my recent book *Innovations: Scientific, Technological and Social* (Oxford University Press, 1970). I have made free use of the many lectures and articles which I have written since *Inventing the Future*, and have quoted myself without quotation marks.

D. G.

London, 17 February 1971

I. A LITTLE DIAGNOSIS OF OUR TIMES

About three-quarters of the population of the globe are still engaged in the age-old occupation of mankind, in the fight against a stingy and hostile Nature. The 'most advanced' quarter has almost defeated Nature, which fights back only as a rotting corpse does; by pollution. In the rich, industrialized countries the fight has turned, almost imperceptibly, into one against human nature.

When in this book I return again and again to the conflict with human nature, I will not forget how nebulous this concept is, and how controversial. I will waste no time in deploring human iniquity and exhorting the sinful people to repent. It would be equally foolish to ignore the weaknesses of human nature. I have little respect for those moral philosophers who, starting with Rousseau, considered Man as intrinsically 'good' and blamed all his evil ways on human institutions. These institutions are themselves logical consequences of human nature, and they have in turn moulded it, by a continuous feedback process which has gone on throughout history. All my hopes and all my fears are in the future of this historical process; how by better social machinery better compromises may be made with an improved human nature. I *believe* in the perfectibility of man, because this is the only working hypothesis for any decent and responsible person. But I *know* of the almost infinite corruptibility of man. History is mostly a sad tale, full of nauseating examples.

My concern in this book is with the 'advanced' quarter of humanity. I certainly do not want to forget the poor three-quarters but I do not agree at all with those men of goodwill who see the solution of our problems in a brotherly sharing of our wealth with them. Rich people at most times have relieved their consciences by charity to the poor. I consider the assistance which we are giving to the poor and struggling countries to be far too small to relieve even a hardened conscience. But let us not indulge in the illusion that even assistance on an adequate scale will solve *our* problems. It may ease, for a while, the problems of the East and of the South, because theirs is the age-old problem of poverty which we in the West have solved by our own efforts, at a terrific cost in human suffering. But our problem has never been solved, because it is new in history and we do not even know whether it can be solved. It is, in brief, the problem of men and women living a peaceful, contented life at a high level of material comfort and security, without the daily struggle for life. If we cannot solve it, what hope can we give to those who are still struggling with our problems of yesterday?

If one wants to give a single name to the troubles which start manifesting themselves in our Western world, I cannot think of anything better than that which Sigmund Freud gave it forty years ago; *The Malaise in Civilisation.** A society in which everybody does only what he likes to do is inconceivable. Any sort of highly developed organization imposes unavoidable constraints on the drives of the individual. These were hated at all times, but the individual's resentment mattered little so long as his actions were forced into a narrow channel by necessity, and also by physical coercion. Slaves and villeins could break out at times in violent revolts, but when these were suppressed with barbaric cruelty, the defeated were forced to accept the old ways of life, however unbearable they appear to us. It was not revolts and revolutions which abolished slavery and serfdom, but the slow, gradual improvement in the means of production, first by the empirical development of the crafts, later by the application of systematic science. This made it possible to establish our liberal democracies which are now in serious danger.

At present we have reached a stage at which the imbalance between facts and expectations favours a destructive outbreak of

---

* *Das Unbehagen in der Kultur*, Vienna, 1930. Translated as *Culture and its Discontents*. The Anglo-French term 'malaise' is a fair equivalent of the German 'Unbehagen'.

the malaise. Freedom from want has been achieved in the industrially advanced countries, not only beyond the dreams of the plague and famine-racked Middle Ages (who in fact hardly dared to dream about a better future), but even beyond the dreams of social reformers fifty years ago. Not of course for everybody, but for the large majority. The 'poverty line' of today is at least equal to the average at the turn of the century. Though much is made, and with full justification, of the relative poverty of the 'underprivileged', it is not the poor minority who threaten us with a revolution of a type with which our society is not prepared to cope. First of all, it is a considerable fraction of the university students. By all standards of the past one would be inclined to consider them as a privileged class; privileged to assimilate the treasures of our culture, which used to be reserved for a small minority. Such a view is of course entirely out of date. It was only the starry-eyed optimism of the utilitarians, such as James Mill and Jeremy Bentham, which could believe that when people have learned to read, they would read the classics, and of course they would be happy ever after! Instead, the malaise in civilization manifests itself most openly on the university campuses. We must not dismiss it lightly because only a small fraction of the students resort to violence, those whom one can classify as emotionally unstable. The 'silent majority' of the students follow their antics with no more than benevolent indifference, but there are good reasons, to which I will return later, for believing that the majority also will soon be seriously disaffected. Nor is there any reason to believe that the disaffected students will settle down, in a few years, to become docile, satisfied members of the consumer society, as most of them have done in the past. This is neither likely, nor is it desirable. The consumer society *must* change into a mature society, and the protest of the young generation is a social force which we must learn to utilize. At its outbreak the student revolt was received with stupefaction, with a wavering between yielding to their 'non-negotiable demands' and repression. Hardly anybody has tried to direct this considerable social force into constructive channels. I believe that this can be done, though only at the cost of reshaping most of the educational process, and many of our values.

A second group which starts behaving militantly are not the poor or the unemployed, but the organized, unionized workers. Strikes have always existed in industrialized countries; they have been outlawed only by the fascists and in the communist third of the world. I would regard them at present as an annoyance rather than as a serious social danger – as a part of the price which we have to pay for a free society. In Britain in recent years, eight to eleven million working days have been lost per year by strikes, which is less than 0.2% of the total, or three to four hours per head per year. Strikes can of course be disruptive far beyond what these figures indicate, because very small groups of workers can throw very large spanners into the intricate machinery of an industrial society. The railwaymen, the seamen, the dockers, the postmen, the lorry drivers, the gas or electricity workers and many others can do serious damage to a whole country. We have seen that even a few hundred upholstery workers can stop the car industry, and throw the delicate foreign trade of a country such as Britain out of balance.* Yet I would not consider industrial disputes to be a revolutionary danger. Several Western countries have survived general strikes without any serious consequences. Georges Sorel may have been right when he described the general strike as the irresistible, ultimate weapon of the working class – but only if there is a revolutionary will behind it, a determination to take over political power. And this determination does not at present exist, not even in countries like Italy and France which have large communist parties. In 1968, in the elections after the student revolts and widespread strikes, the French Communist Party posed as the party of law and order. These communist parties now live and prosper by what Freud has called 'goal-inhibited drives'. They are not at all keen on reaching their goal, which is a socialist country such as the USSR, where there are no strikes and no protests, and where revolutionaries are soon replaced by *apparatchiki*.

What I consider a more important symptom of things to come than industrial disputes is *silent* protest; the spreading of voluntary absenteeism in most industrialized countries. It has started in Britain and has spread to France and Italy, and to the United

* See Note 1.

States. Only Germany and Japan seem to be immune to it for the time being. In Britain it is estimated to have caused the loss of between 300 and 400 million working days per year, which is at least thirty, but perhaps forty, times more than have been lost by strikes. It varies widely between different industries, it is about 2% in the electrical industry, almost 20% in mining. On the whole the loss is about 5 to 6·5% of the total working time, which is sufficient to make all the difference between a good rate of growth and stagnation.* In Italy voluntary absenteeism was negligible until the law was abolished under which the firm had the right to send a doctor to absent workers. Three days later absenteeism in the Alfa-Romeo works in Turin jumped from 6% to 18%. In the United States it has also become a serious cause for worry. In Detroit the voluntary absenteeism on Mondays is of the order of 5% to 10%, caused mostly by young workers. It is likely to increase steadily as the older workers are gradually replaced by the younger, who have greater expectations of what they are entitled to receive from life. In the USA absenteeism has been tackled by symptomatic remedies, such as rewards for good attendance, also by experiments with a 4-day, 40-hour week. The first has failed already, the second is certain to fail, in spite of initial successes.†

I have brought voluntary absenteeism into focus as an important industrial ailment of our times, not so much because of its economic significance, but because it is a clear symptom of the revolt against the consumer society. The voluntary under-consumption of the workers who exchange a part of their pay for free time seems to me more impressive than the rather histrionic 'conspicuous underconsumption' of the students and hippies in their pre-patched jeans. Ostensibly, the industrial disputes are always for more pay, but a not insignificant minority of the workers prefer less work for less pay. They are not afraid of the boredom of leisure; even a Monday in a Welsh mining village appears preferable to the boredom of a day at the coalface. There is of course no boredom when the workers go hunting or fishing,

---

* The real figure may be even higher if one adds to it a fraction of 'certified sickness'. See Note 2.

† See Note 3.

but even if there is nothing much to fill their free time, it is sweetened by the feeling that it is an expression of *protest*, the satisfaction of having damaged a little the hated industrial machinery, and of having followed their own free will.

So long as this phenomenon remains within moderate limits, one can consider it a safety valve for the expression of social dissatisfaction, which it would be dangerous to tie down. I am even inclined to view it as a hopeful signpost towards a mature society. If workers are happy with their poor, purse-pinched leisure, we can expect them to be even happier when they are educated to enjoy leisure. But in the transition period this silent protest can lead to serious difficulties.

In the communist countries, where strikes are illegal, the continual monotonous work leads to dull boredom, a 'couldn't-care-less' attitude on the part of the workers, who become even more effectively alienated than the workers in the capitalist countries. Nevertheless, production (though still on a low level) has steadily increased in the USSR in the years when it has come almost to a standstill in the USA and in Britain, and herein lies a danger. The expectation of growth is the chief driving power in the free economies, and now, paradoxically, this is seriously endangered by the 'revolution of expectations' of the workers, coupled with the signs of saturation. Getting more for less work was by no means an impossibility so long as technological progress steadily increased the productivity per man-hour. But the expectation of reduced or even zero growth in production and consumption naturally slows down the investment rate, which has already fallen to a dangerously low level in the USA and in Britain. If the gap between expectations and productive investments widens, the outcome will be either a crash, with unemployment, bankruptcies and such a low standard of living that the incentives of poverty will come into action again, as they have so often done in the past, or else there will be an irresistible temptation for governments to follow the example of the more stable totalitarian countries, taking over a much larger sector of the economy and further restricting private initiative and personal freedom.

What is even more dangerous and more likely is that the

totalitarian governments, seeing the difficulties of liberal-democratic systems, will slow down or stop the process of liberalization, the convergence of our system and theirs, which not so long ago was one of our great white hopes. It is so much easier to govern a nation which is not too rich, not too free; why then give up the spirit of the garrison-state and produce more consumer goods instead of more armaments?*

This must not happen. The weaknesses of our liberal-democratic system must not encourage the totalitarian rulers to tighten the reins, and to throw their dynamism into an expansionist tendency. One of my chief preoccupations in this book is the conflict between social stability and personal freedom. I regard freedom, the right of the individual to follow his will, as a value in itself, and a certain degree of disorder and conflict as not too high a price to pay for it. But in the past personal freedom has also been a mighty force for social improvement. I would like to see as much of it as possible harnessed for the great transformation of society which is before us. 'Harness' and 'freedom' are not a hopeless contradiction. There remains a wide range for free individual choice even after excluding anti-social actions. It was this limited freedom which, in the past, brought vast economic success to the democratic countries as against the old, bigoted autocracies. The situation has changed now, the new autocracies are also 'democratic' in the sense that they have no hereditary dynasties and ruling classes, but they are not liberal. They suffer no political opposition and no free press, not even a free literature. Their idea of social stability is to clamp down on every manifestation of personal freedom and criticism. This is undeniably a safe

---

* Optimistic readers will probably hold against me that at the 24th Party Congress, 1971, the Soviets have again announced a great increase in consumer goods in the new Five Year Plan. I wish that I could believe that this will be at the expense of armaments. What makes me doubtful is the statement that the increase of investment in the steel industry (70% above that of the last five years) is twice that of the average over all industries. Steel production is to be built up to nearly 150 million tons per year, which is about equal to the US capacity, but far in excess of US production. How much of this will go into consumer goods? Even assuming that the target of 800,000 private motor cars per annum is reached by the end of the next period, this would amount to rather less than *one per cent* of the steel output.

way, so long as it is combined with a reasonable degree of efficiency. Talleyrand may have been right: one cannot sit for ever safely on bayonets; but the modern tyrants, far more purposeful and watchful than those of the Holy Alliance, can sit on them for a very long time. Our liberal democracies will be in great danger when the psychological ailment, of which I have so far listed two symptoms, spreads and impregnates the masses with fear; they will then notice that superior efficiency is no longer on our side, and they may be willing to barter their freedom for safety.

Two more of the unhealthy symptoms of our times must be mentioned. One is the frightening increase in drug addiction, the other is the mounting level of crime. The two are closely connected because the drug epidemic, at any rate in the United States, is largely the work of organized crime. But why does it find so many willing victims, who are ready to sacrifice their health for an escape into a dream world? The propensity has probably always been present, and in all classes. In 18th-century Britain it was not only the gin-sodden proletarians who regularly got dead drunk; so did the Anglo-Irish gentry.* Perhaps it was not so much education and improvement in the quality of life which reduced alcoholism, but the cigarette. It is very probable that if the present strong drive against tobacco were successful, alcoholism and drug addiction would again show a strong increase, unless a harmless substitute is found. Prohibition in the United States was the most resounding failure of an idealistically inspired social experiment in all history, and it is not likely to be repeated with tobacco. I do not think that drug addiction rises because there are more escapists in our world than in the past, but there is much more temptation and opportunity. One can foresee that the fight against drugs will be a never-ending struggle. We shall be able to call ourselves lucky if the civilization of the future can co-exist with the new, chemically produced drugs, as our Western civilization has in the past co-existed with alcohol. The probable

* That opportunity is more important than propensity is confirmed by the sad fact that the social group with by far the greatest fraction of drug addicts are doctors and nurses – a group with a moral fibre certainly stronger than the average.

alternatives are either a new, harmless drug like Aldous Huxley's 'Soma', or else a society closely supervized by the police. Note that drugs have been fairly efficiently suppressed in the USSR, and opium almost completely in Red China.

The steep increase of crime in the Western societies was and is a deep shock for all liberals, who believed that crime was a by-product of poverty and ignorance. For some time many well-meaning people doubted the statistical figures, and attributed them to better methods of detection. But in recent years the statistics have become so frightening, and so many people had personal experience of it as victims, that it must be recognized as a major social danger. The figures for Britain speak for themselves.

	TOTAL CRIMES	VIOLENCE	BURGLARY AND ROBBERY
1930	147,031	2,123	25,937
1940	305,114	2,424	49,339
1950	461,713	6,249	92,839
1960	743,713	15,759	151,378
1969	1,427,294	32,654	414,894
1970	1,560,000	37,000	470,000

The doubling of crimes for gain between 1930 and 1940 may be attributable to the great slump, but the fifteenfold increase of violence between 1940 and 1970 defies such a simple materialistic explanation. It is a manifestation of human nature at its worst, at its most unrestrained, greedy for 'kicks'. It is time to take it very seriously, and not just by multiplying prisons and strengthening the police forces.

I have listed here four symptoms of the malaise in civilization which manifest themselves in some of the most advanced free Western countries: the revolt of the university youth, voluntary absenteeism, drug addiction and crime. I have listed them together, but they are on very different moral levels. The first two contain an element of hope. The revolt of the university youth is fed by idealism; in the United States it takes its main strength from the very justified revulsion against the Vietnam war. At present its manifestations are mostly negative, its strongest feature is villain-hunting, but the enthusiasm which often goes to the point of self-sacrifice is a valuable social force which it must be possible to enlist for much-needed reform. The silent protest which manifests itself in voluntary absenteeism also contains an element of hope; it seems to show that there may be less resistance than one might have expected to slowing down the whirling-dervish economy of the consumer society.

These two groups contain an element of hope, but it must be mentioned that they also have a disturbing feature in common. Both offer an opportunity for troublemakers, for small minorities who can create disturbances in society disproportionate to their numbers, and whose goals are often only excuses for the satisfaction which they find in the act of rebellion itself.

Drug addiction and crime are truly pathological symptoms, which increasingly affect the weakest and the worst members of our rich and free society. The young rebels would of course passionately deny that it is free, but it is free compared to the totalitarian societies which are also less rich, and in which all these four ills are cured by the simple method of repression.

There may be 'symptomatic' cures for these ills, other than simple repression, but there is only one general remedy: *the love of life*. Unfortunately, human nature is such that it loves life best when it is in danger. It was this basic feature which made our ancestors survive plagues, famines and wars. I have no doubt that it will make our descendants survive, much reduced in numbers and chastened, even the worst catastrophes which we are preparing in our folly – even a nuclear war. We are now at an 'up' in history, the highest ever reached; can we prevent another 'down'? Can we create a society worthy of being loved, and can we make men and women love life when it is secure? These are the problems to which I will address myself in this book, in the hope that others will follow me.

2. THE WORLD SCENE

In the economically successful free countries we are suffering from the aimless confusion which follows our undigested technical victory. Dangerous social tensions have developed, which can only be overcome either by repression, or by a purposeful, planned transformation towards a better society. But can we risk such a transformation in a hostile environment? There are many people among us, and not just members of the military-industrial complex, who fear that if we direct our efforts inwards, towards a more humane, more just, society, we shall be destroyed by the monolithic giants. Nobody can say in good conscience that these fears are illusory. We know that nobody could put his head into the lap of Stalin, and since the invasion of Czechoslovakia we also know that it would be dangerous to try this with the lap of Brezhnev. The danger exists, but fear is a bad counsellor. Let us try to take an objective view of the power game which is now being played out in the less developed, poorer parts of the world – a playground which at any moment could change into a battleground.

This game is sharply distinguished from the struggle for colonies in past centuries. Colonies could be exploited, and could (though not always did) add to the wealth of the colonizer. Today it has become a strictly zero-sum game between the great powers, where the gain of one is the loss of the other. The United States have not sent a costly expedition to Vietnam in order to exploit that poor peasant country. The USSR have not sent many billion dollars worth of arms and military assistance to the Arab countries in order to get hold of their oil, which they do not use, and do not need. All such moves are directed against the opponent in the power game; the country where they take place is at most a pawn.

I consider that these moves are to a great extent *compulsive*, not so much parts of a grand design, or products of the will of the rulers, as forced on them by fear and by the power situations in their own country which they control only imperfectly. We *know* that the United States has no political master plan to destroy the Socialist Republics. But neither do I believe that the incessant stirring up of trouble by the USSR in one quarter of the world after another is part of a grand design for world domination, and for destroying the United States. Undoubtedly, these are all hostile moves against the USA but they are prompted far more by a largely irrational *fear* than by a steely will towards world domination. If any of the great powers ever dominated the 'world', this would consist only of radioactive (perhaps virus-infected) smoking ruins, and I do not believe that either the USA or the USSR are ruled by paranoid schizophrenics.

The power game is, to use Freud's illuminating term, 'goal-inhibited', but nevertheless I expect it to go on lustily for a long time, simply because there are so many potential trouble-spots in the world where intervention by the great powers will be almost automatic. After Cuba and Vietnam the Middle East, perhaps again Korea, perhaps Africa, Latin-America. . . . Any change of power, any insurgency in any far corner of the world, will jangle nerves in Washington and in Moscow. (However, after the collapse of the Vietnam adventure it may not lead so easily to a military intervention.) In all probability this nervous tension will remain a permanent feature for the rest of the 20th century, and it can break out at any moment in smaller or larger wars.

But not in an all-out nuclear or biological war between the US and the USSR! When, like almost everybody else, I base my predictions and suggestions on this assumption, I believe that I am on solid ground. If we look around us, we can see that this is also the 'working hypothesis' adopted by peoples and by govern-ments alike. Few parents are afraid of bringing children into this world, in which they could be wiped out in a nuclear war, because in their heart they do not believe in its possibility. If governments really believed in it, they would have to proclaim an emergency, take draconic measures for the dispersion of the population and of industry, set armies of workers building deep shelters, and put the power and water systems and huge stocks of food and fuel underground. Only peaceful Sweden has done this to any considerable extent. Instead of this, governments only weakly oppose the crowding together of the population in huge conurbations, they have their food and fuel stocks above ground, and they allow the systems for the distribution of power and water to be so weak as to work most of the time near the limit of their capacity, with frequent breakdowns. In brief, they have resisted hardly at all the natural tendency of all industrial countries to become more and more vulnerable.

The USA and the USSR have put their efforts not into defence but into deterrence. The ABM (Anti-Ballistic Missile) system in the United States has the purpose of 'hardening' the deterrence, by protecting the missile sites, so that they shall be able to deliver the counterstrike. This has been done in the USA against the advice of almost every scientist who is not a member of the establishment, but they were overruled when the USSR foolishly started with it. The ABM, both in the USA and in the USSR, is a typical compulsive measure. The everlasting fear finds its outlet on the path of least resistance, where there is a small pretence of usefulness, but a very real benefit for the armaments establishment. (In the USSR the armaments industry is not a clearly defined profit-making body, but it is nonetheless an establishment, with enormous pressure.) This fateful step has been taken, though hardly anybody in the USA seriously believes (or even professes to believe), that the Soviets will one night launch an all-out nuclear attack under the protection of their very leaky ABM umbrella. In the USSR there are people who pretend to believe in a Pearl Harbor of the USA. Their staff journals publish at regular intervals 'reliable' reports from their agents about an impending devastating attack by the USA against the Socialist Republics. But I just cannot believe that anybody, perhaps least of all a highly trained Russian Staff officer, could believe that a mad American President, short-circuiting all the constitutional safeguards, could one night give the order for the mutual suicide of his country and of the USSR, and that he would be obeyed.

Summing up the whole situation, I would give a nuclear or biological war between the USA and the USSR in this century the probability *nil*. I fear there can be no such certainty as regards the USSR and China. It is not true that we occidentals cannot understand the Chinese mentality. I believe that we can perfectly well understand them *individually*; they are people like us. But it is unfortunately true that the web of constraints under which the Chinese live has created a *public* mentality which is beyond our understanding. Thousands of years of autocratic rule have made the Chinese masters in the art of not saying what they think, but saying what they think is expected from them. Pragmatism, in an extreme form. On the rather rare occasions when Western scientists had an opportunity to talk about world affairs with Chinese scientists, they were extremely disturbed and depressed by their paranoiac-sounding statements. They simply repeated, parrot-fashion, that China cannot be defeated in a nuclear war. They may yet have to pay dearly for this egregious conventional lie. I cannot believe that they *wish* for a nuclear war, but they might provoke it if they continue to build up their missile strength and accompany this with threats and vituperations until they strain the nerves of Moscow beyond the breaking-point.

Our best hope is, as always, the great panacea: *time*. If we survive some decades of tension without an explosion, the tension will subside, as it did in Western Europe, though only after many centuries of war. In the past sobering has only come after horrible devastation. But history need not always repeat itself. We need not play forever the zero-sum game in an epoch in which science pays so much better than war. Perhaps the Chinese will in time build up a great, rich, civilized empire within their own vast frontiers, without having first to suffer a devastating defeat.

Let us have no illusions; the advanced, rich countries of the world will have to take the first steps towards maturity in a world full of trouble, under constant nervous tension. We cannot change this situation from one day to the next, we must write it into our calculations for a long time. With patience and wisdom we may be able to reduce international tension gradually, and break the fatal feedback loop of fear. Unless we can do this, we will not only build costly Maginot Lines with imaginary usefulness, but there will be the constant danger of frightened rulers scaring their flock into an acceptance of authoritarianism. If we take the right path, maturity itself will reduce the tension, and during the time of the transformation, the tension may help to make it maturity without decadence. The great creative epochs – Periclean Greece, the Italy of the Renaissance, Elizabethan England, France at the time of the Revolution – were epochs of tension and danger.

3. CAPITALISM, TECHNOLOGY AND GROWTH

The bourgeoisie during its rule of scarce one hundred years has created more massive and more colossal productive forces than have all preceding generations together. Subjection of nature's forces to man, machinery, application of chemistry to industry and agriculture, steam-navigation, railways, electric telegraphs, clearing of whole continents for cultivation, canalization of rivers, whole populations conjured out of the ground – what earlier century had even a presentiment that such productive forces slumbered in the lap of social labour?

(*The Communist Manifesto*, 1848)

This fine compliment was paid by Marx and Engels to their enemies. It may be somewhat surprising that they wrote 'bourgeoisie' where we would say 'science and technology', but they saw something we can easily miss. We take it for granted that our social system makes full use of technology, but they saw perhaps more clearly than we that it was the rise of capitalism which had accomplished 'wonders far surpassing Egyptian pyramids, Roman aqueducts and Gothic cathedrals' – the achievements of the feudal and monolithic systems of the past. They would have been dismayed to know that their powerful battle-cry would lead to a monolithic system, which, at any rate up to the present day, is less efficient than capitalism.

Let us take stock of what capitalism has achieved, in the 120-odd years after the *Manifesto*, in that most capitalistic of all countries, in the United States. Let us first examine material goods, which can be expressed in numbers.

In 1970, of 63 million families, 64% owned their own houses –

50% even of those below the poverty line of $3000 p.a., who numbered 6·3 million, or 10% of the population. They owned 104 million private cars – even of the families below the poverty line 41% owned one car; on the whole 29·3% of the families had at least two cars. The list of other consumer durables is no less impressive: 99·8% of all families owned refrigerators, 95% at least one television set, 37·8% at least one colour set, 29·4% more than one set; 91·9% owned washing machines, 40·3% clothes dryers, 36·7% air conditioners, 29·6% freezers, 23·7% dishwashers.* It can be seen that saturation in consumer durables, that is to say a state in which gadgets have only to be replaced when they have worn out, cannot be far away.

The Americans are also rich in goods which cannot be so easily measured by statistics. The overwhelming majority of the workers have clean well-dressed wives, strong healthy children, and few of them, if any, have ever experienced hunger; not even those below the poverty line of $3000 per family, which is at least five to eight times more than the average in the under-developed third of the world. It is also at least equal to the average income per family in the USSR or in any other communist country, measured in terms of real consumption and not in the easily manipulated 'GNP per capita'. Even allowing for the devaluation of money, it would have been a 'bourgeois' income at the time of the *Communist Manifesto*.

This book is essentially a critique of our system and its tendencies, therefore it behoves the critic to pay as great a tribute to the positive achievements of mature capitalism as Marx and Engels have paid to its ruthless adolescent ancestor.

But the Americans are far from happy. Everybody is worried about inflation, quite a few about the possibility of unemployment. Even those older people who feel fairly secure in their well-paid jobs, and who can still remember the misery of the great slump in the thirties, are for the most part greatly worried about their children, who are protesting increasingly against the values of the 'achievement-oriented society'.

The belief in the simple values of work and fair reward for

* Corresponding figures in the United Kingdom were, in 1969, 60% refrigerators, 63% washing machines, 51% cars.

work, achieved by an ever-improving technology, used nowhere to be stronger than in the United States, where it has now suffered the strongest set-back. 'Stagflation' (stagnation *cum* inflation) had a worse psychological impact on the Americans than on any other people, because they had counted on automatic, year-to-year growth more than anybody else. The draconian measures which President Nixon had to introduce in August 1971 have driven it home even to the most complacent, that the recession which started in 1968 would not blow over by itself without an unusual degree of state intervention. For many this was a rude awakening from the 'American Dream'. They were also hit, though less badly, by the sudden realization of the dangerously increasing level of pollution. In simple terms this means that the USA, like most industrial countries, has lived beyond its means by not spending enough on the elimination of waste products. I will not discuss pollution at length, because it could be mastered in the USA as elsewhere by spending about 1·5% of the GNP, and this figure could remain fairly constant to the end of the century. It would not impede economic growth, it means only a once-for-all tightening of the belt. Let us realize that our system is only 98·5% as efficient as we imagined, and deal with it! I am far more concerned about the psychological components in the crisis of industrial civilization, which are receiving much less attention.

Next to the United States, Britain has been worst hit by inflation and stagnation, with its attendant economic troubles. That the psychological upset is less than in the States is probably mainly due to the fact that growth was never quite the fetish in the UK it was in the USA. But for the same reason, the malady will probably be more difficult to cure. Voluntary absenteeism, the unwillingness to work more or harder, is more prominent in Britain than perhaps anywhere else; it is not without reason that it has been called on the Continent 'the English disease'.

At the time of writing, Germany and Japan are still free of this disease. It is no accident that these are the two countries which were almost entirely destroyed in the war. Scrambling up from the bottom appears to be a difficult exercise, but it is one for which the human race, and especially such able and energetic people as the Germans and the Japanese, are singularly well equipped. But it cannot be very many years before they too, after having triumphantly overcome 'growing pains', will be faced by what I would call the 'pains of maturing'.

In this book, as in my previous writings, I am taking a determined stand on the thesis that growth will have to reach a turning-point and that we must work towards a gentle saturation, or, as others would say, towards a stable ecosystem. This is easily misunderstood, or perhaps consciously misinterpreted, by those who accuse us 'anti-growth heretics' of wanting to stop growth here and now. Nothing could be more misleading. Growth is a many-faceted amd multidimensional phenomenon, it has its healthy and unhealthy sides. Let us look first at some trends and potentialities.

There is first of all the population growth. Everybody knows that it will have to come to a stop some time, because the area and the resources of the world are finite. My contention is that it ought to be brought to a stop long before the Malthusian limit is reached, which some authorities put as high as 15 to 45 thousand million people. Existential nausea will make the giant cities of the future highly explosive long before that. But we cannot stop population growth overnight. Demographers* have calculated that even if all couples in the USA were to adopt tomorrow the exact replacement rate of 2·25 children, the population would still grow for about sixty years to a level of about 280 million before the stationary state is reached, simply because there are now so many young couples.† It is true that the example of Hungary has shown that free abortion can make the reproduction rate drop not only below the replacement rate, but also below the mortality rate, but this was an exceptional phenomenon, which

* Larry Bumpass and Charles F. Westoff, *The Perfect Contraceptive Population*, Science, **169**, 18 September 1970, p. 1177. A survey made by these authors has led to the interesting conclusion that almost 20% of the births in the USA are unwanted, and their elimination would reduce reproduction to close to the replacement rate. The estimate by the Health Education Council of unwanted births in Britain is 120,000, which is about 13·5%.

† At the time of writing a surprising drop is reported in the US birth rate, which makes it appear possible that the maximum might be reached in this century. But it is more likely a transient effect of the recession.

lasted only for a few years. We must resign ourselves to the fact that a stationary state will not be reached in the industrial countries in less than fifty years perhaps, and in the underdeveloped countries, short of major catastrophes, a few decades later, by which time the world population will be hardly less than 8 thousand million. This will be a time of crisis, whatever we do.

Second, there is industrial growth. The food industry *must* grow faster than world population, because about half of the world's population are suffering from an insufficient and monotonous diet, which can arrest not only their physical but also their mental development below the point at which they can be expected to restrict their reproduction rate from a feeling of social responsibility, and not because of starvation. The know-how is available; dwarf wheat, hybrid maize and high-yield rice may be able to feed a world population two to three times the present figure. All these, however, require an enormous increase in the use of fertilizers. Nitrogen can be obtained from the air, but I have nowhere found any assurance that the still vast deposits of potash and phosphates will last much longer than perhaps a hundred years. It is useless to worry about this now, because it is an ethical imperative that we must feed the world population with the means at our disposal, and feed it well. We could not do otherwise, even if it were proved beyond any doubt that a hundred-odd years hence we shall have reached the Malthusian limit.

Industrial development in the poor third or half of the world presents us with a similar dilemma. It is extremely unlikely that these nations could be brought up to the American or Western European level of consumption within thirty or even fifty years. If they were, some of the key metals and minerals would be exhausted well within the next hundred years. Recently attention has been drawn to another danger. The pollution per inhabitant in the upper fifth of the world is about fifty times more than that in the other four-fifths, and full industrial development might raise the world pollution rate to a level at which it might kill off the major part of the world's population (as will be shown later in some interesting computer simulations of the future). The danger is probably smaller than suggested by these terrifying forecasts, because industry in the underdeveloped countries will not grow so fast, but it is serious enough. If we in the leading industrial countries find it so difficult to raise the 1·5% of the GNP needed to suppress pollution, how much worse will it be in the developing countries, who cannot afford to bother about such niceties?

The situation in the advanced countries is fundamentally different. We too have our difficulties, which can be classed, in increasing order of importance, as technological, institutional and psychological. They form an interwoven complex, but for a start let us single out the easiest, the one which gives the widest limits: technology. We follow a procedure similar to that which the navy uses when it is looking for an enemy ship which has been sighted at a certain spot at a certain time. It must then be inside a circle, drawn with a radius which it could have sailed in a straight line, at maximum speed. Let us see how far technology could take us by the year 2000 in the absence of countervailing forces.

About 150 years ago 80% of the population had to work the land, in order to provide just enough food for all. (This is still the proportion in China.) In fact it was not even sufficient – most of the population was stunted. Even in England a good inch was added to the height of the sons of the working classes when, during and after the war, they enjoyed for the first time a varied and plentiful diet. In the United States, at the time of writing, about 5% of the labour force produce more than enough food not only for the 200 million Americans (of whom millions are weight watchers, who daily send many thousand tons of uneaten food down the drain), but for scores of millions abroad, and are heavily subsidized for not growing more. Fifteen years ago it was still a little more than 10% of the labour force, and a reasonable projection indicates that by 1982 it will be only 2·5%.

What has happened in agriculture can happen in all production industries. The technological development which makes this possible is usually called by the vogue word 'automation'. In its strict sense this term ought to be reserved for the so-called 'cybernetic' machines, which have some sort of sensory organ, so that they 'know what they are doing'. As a simple example, an automatic lathe in which the tool is set to some nominal measure is not cybernetic. The measure may be wrong because of wear on the tool, or because of the elasticity of the job. On the other hand a lathe which has a continuously measuring organ, which indicates the true measure and sets the tool so that it shall produce the desired value, is a cybernetic machine, with 'sensory feedback'. This is an old invention of Nature; we are all cybernetic machines when we control the writing hand by the eye. It is not new in engineering either (James Watt's centrifugal governor will soon be 200 years old), but the idea has undergone an enormous extension and refinement in the past forty years. *Any* machine, automaton or robot which is to compete with human beings in jobs requiring intelligence, will have to be cybernetic. But the present economic importance of such devices need not be over-rated. Mechanization and rationalization of processes are still by far the most important ways of saving human labour. As an example, containerization of freight can save 90% of the dockers and also 70% of the crews and ships, owing to the rapid turn-round. In the Appalachian mines mechanization has reduced the number of coal miners from 530,000 to 140,000, little over a quarter. A similar reduction has been achieved in the UK in the last twenty years. The reduction in the number of road-workers from the time when it was done by navvies with spades and wheelbarrows is near to 99%. These were all jobs requiring little intelligence, and what intelligence is needed can now be supplied by *one* operator of a bulldozer or drag-line.

At the present time in the USA 'manual' or 'blue-collar' workers (both terms have become rather metaphoric) make up only one-third of the labour force, in the European industrial countries about one-half of it. The proportion is steadily sinking in all industries, while the total labour force remains a remarkably constant fraction of the population. (In the USA about 39% are gainfully employed in civilian occupations, in the UK and in Germany about 47%.) The rest are busy in offices, in service occupations and in the professions.

How far can this proportion decrease by AD 2000? A straight extrapolation of the last five to ten years gives about 20% for the USA, about 40% for the UK. But these are extrapolations of the reductions obtained in the face of constant opposition by the labour unions. If we are interested in what technological progress *could* achieve if it were unopposed, we can accept the estimate by US automation experts that the blue-collar labour force could decrease by half a million a year, instead of increasing by one and a half million, and this gives about 10% by AD 2000, assuming that the total labour force remains a fairly constant fraction of the population. In the UK the difference between the extrapolated and the potential decrease is even larger. On the whole 2·5 workmen are employed in Britain for the production of one man in the States. If by some miracle the *present* efficiency of the USA could be achieved in Britain, the fraction of manual production workers could at once drop to 20%.

I must repeat that I am not talking of *expected* figures. The resistance of the labour unions will not cease, and this is just as well so long as we do not know what to do with the 'technological unemployment'. I am seeking only to show that by the end of the century technology, if given a free hand, could bring about as dramatic a reduction of all 'manual' labour as we have already experienced in agriculture. Other authorities have arrived at even lower figures by assuming that the major part of the production will be done in fully automated factories.

But are there no limits set to the efficiency of technology by the exhaustion of raw materials? We are steadily depleting the natural supplies of metals, coal, oil and natural gas, though for the last fifty years the progress in prospecting has been such that the proven reserves have always grown instead of decreasing. Will there not be a time when scraping together the metal supply from low-grade ores will set a limit to progress? Only a few years ago the answer might have been doubtful, though even then one could confidently predict that there would be no crisis before the end of the century. But some time oil, and also oil shale, will be exhausted, and carburants will have to be produced artificially. Though there are enough metals in the Earth's crust and in the seas, they occur only in a highly diluted form, and their separation requires immense expenditure of energy. Eight years ago, when I wrote my first book, controlled fusion was the only hope for an abundant source of power which could not be exhausted by humanity, however extravagant, in a million years. In the meantime this hope has almost faded out, but technological progress has replaced it by two solid realities. Uranium is present in the rocks and the seas in immense quantities. It has proved economical to grind down granite and separate the uranium, which may be only 0·1 to 0·3%, at a cost of only about twice that of uranium from high-grade ores. In the long run it will be even more important that uranium can be extracted from the seas, in which it is dissolved with a concentration of only 3 milligrams per cubic metre, at probably not more than four times the present world price. This reservoir can never be exhausted, because the rivers wash more uranium into the seas each year than could be consumed by a world population several times the present, and fully industrialized. There is therefore no danger of industrial civilization ever coming to an end through shortage of power, and with abundant power all metals can be extracted, even from the poorest deposits, or from the sea. I am rather more doubtful about fertilizers, because recovering phosphorus from its highly dilute solution in the seas at anything like reasonable cost is still a problem beyond present-day chemistry. But this is not yet a problem of the near future.

Let us now turn to other dimensions. Medical science has already extended the life expectation at birth in the industrial countries to over 70 years, in spite of smoking, pollution and road accidents, but for the older people it is usually not much better than 'medicated survival'. It is not too much to expect that by the end of the century science will restore for the older people, if not youthful vigour, at least the health and strength of the prime of life. This is more important than an extension of the life span by, say, twenty years, and also more likely.

Technology can even solve an apparently impossible problem; providing more unspoilt Nature, more green fields and forests for an increased population. The new crops, such as the new strain of rice, are so economical that only a fraction of the area now under cultivation would be needed even in seemingly over-populated countries, like India. (The modern methods of meat production, such as broiler chickens and battery calves are even more economical in area, if rather barbarous.) But even greater progress can be expected from the growing of micro-organisms on oil, in the sea and in tanks, ultimately even from the synthesis of edible proteins. For my part I would prefer a population feeding on steak and pheasants, but fully as tasty substitutes are not out of the question. It would then be possible to concentrate food production in a restricted area and let men do with the rest as they like best. Make it into gardens and parks, surrounding large family houses, or leave the land in its more or less natural state, where the city population can enjoy their holidays in an environment better suited to their instincts.* At present, it must be admitted, we are going in the opposite direction; industrialization destroys the beauty spots of the world instead of adding to them. But at least we have become aware of the problem, and the conservationists have grown to a powerful pressure group.

I started by extrapolating the achievements of present-day technology; in the case of unspoilt nature I have come to an example where it starts defeating itself. This is even more obvious in the case of rapid transport, which has made the world not only small, but too small. In 1970 six million Britons enjoyed holidays abroad, mostly in the sunshine of France, Spain and Italy. There is no technical, or even fundamental economic hindrance to this number growing to, say, 30 million, and not just for two weeks per year, but for four or more. Improved production methods could pay for their holidays, and jet planes (with a great organizational effort, involving many more airports) could take them there, but will it be worth their while if they line the sea coast in deckchairs eight or ten rows deep, and feed in cafeterias, probably automated? Those who ask for nothing more than sunshine may perhaps be satisfied, but those who want to see beautiful old towns and works of art will be frustrated. Venice or Florence can hardly take twice the present number of tourists, let alone ten times.† The aristocratic beauties of the past cannot be democratically shared by all. This is a problem technology cannot solve. It

---

* See Nigel Calder, *The Environment Game*, Secker & Warburg, London, 1967.

† L. Tončič-Sorinj, Secretary General of the Council of Europe: 'Tourism not only feeds on our cultural heritage, it is liable to destroy it utterly.'

can give the masses food, clothing, shelter, travel and entertainment, but in the end it cannot by itself avoid giving them some frustration also.

Still, let us not belittle science and technology because they cannot give us *everything*. Would we exchange the embarrassment of riches for the poverty of the past when life was poor, nasty, brutish and short? Certainly only those of us who imagine that they would have been aristocrats! The democratic Utopia which technology can give us may not be very attractive, but the alternatives are much worse.

4.   UTOPIA AND REALITY

The sketch on the limits of material development outlined in the previous chapter is completely realistic in terms of the scientific-technological possibilities, completely unrealistic if we take into consideration the present state of the world and the present moral development of Man. In its riches it is far beyond the dreams of any of the early Utopians, but we no longer believe in Utopias. What are the reasons for this sad change? One is, certainly, that in this century we have lived through two terrible world wars of a ferocity which might well have shaken even the belief of a Jeremy Bentham in the perfectibility of man. But the other, and probably the more important reason is that we have also seen an epoch of unparalleled material progress – without any enthusiasm or pride. The standard of living has at least doubled in all industrial countries. When my Italian house was built (in which I write these lines) the workmen all came in their little Fiat cars. Before the war they would have come on bicycles or on foot. Yet unrest in Italy is as strong as it ever was. Perhaps Schumpeter was right when he wrote: 'Secular improvement that is taken for granted and coupled with individual insecurity that is acutely resented is of course the best recipe to breed social unrest.'[*] I think most of our contemporaries would consider these lines, written twenty years ago, as unduly optimistic, because they imply that one has only to remove individual insecurity to make the people happy. I am rather inclined to believe that complete material security, from the cradle to the grave, would be the best

[*] Joseph A. Schumpeter, *Capitalism and Democracy*, 3rd ed., Harper Brothers, New York, 1950, p. 145.

recipe to create unbearable boredom and bring out the worst in Irrational Man. Especially when he can have all the security and the material comforts with that minimum of work which is sufficient in a highly developed technological society.

It was easy for Edward Bellamy, the most practical and inventive of Utopian writers, to paint the picture of a glorious Boston against the background of the poverty-ridden city of 1888. Today most of what he dreamed has been realized, even the sample store with punched vouchers, and the radio; unlimited good music for everybody. One must admit though that in one respect we have fallen sadly behind his dream. Where is the collective pride? In his Boston of AD 2000 'Every quarter contained large open squares filled with trees, along which statues glistened and fountains flashed in the late afternoon sun. Public buildings of a colossal size and architectural grandeur unparalleled in my time raised their stately piles on every side.' The modern Boston has rather less of this grandeur than the old. Yet would people be free from individual unrest even if these stately palaces were dedicated to the most humanitarian tasks, to the administration of Assistance, Medicare and Medicaid? Not with people as they are at present!

The American people have just passed the threshold of what Herman Kahn called the 'Post-industrial Society' with $4000 GNP per capita, and are on the way to its upper limit at $20,000, beyond which comes the 'Post-economic Society'.* I do not think that these upper figures have much meaning. Only the most naïve can imagine that they would be able to have the sort of life which people with such an income are enjoying at present. 'Money alone does not make for happiness' used to be hypocritical advice when given to the poor. It becomes sober reality when applied to the rich, especially when everybody is rich.

In all the past thousand years of civilization, people who had to work longed to be free of it, and envied the privileged who did not have to work for their living. The Good Fairy, Technology, is now mocking us with the fulfilment of this ancestral wish. The Age of Leisure is staring us in the face. We are still defending ourselves against it by stretching the economy of

* See Note 4.

scarcity beyond its natural limits, by restrictive practices and by Parkinson's Law.

The reduction of the productive labour required for a given output has been with us for a long time. It has accelerated since the war to such an extent that the 'blue-collar' labour force has actually decreased in the USA and in the Western countries, though the populations increased at the rate of 1 to 2% p.a. and the consumption per capita by 2 to 6%. Still unemployment remained in reasonable limits, from 2 to 6%, while the total labour force increased in almost exactly the same proportion as the population. (It now shows a tendency to increase somewhat more rapidly, owing to the post-war 'bulge' in births, which made more young people available.) How have we dealt with the labour which has become redundant on the production lines? Chiefly by sending it into the offices.

In the United States, at the time of writing, unemployment is kept at a level of 4 to 6% by keeping $2\frac{1}{2}$ million young men under arms, by a major war in Vietnam, by an enormous war industry, but chiefly by Parkinson's Law. The American economy could manage without the Vietnam war, but the alternative would be to increase civilian consumption much more steeply. In 1966 an important national commission estimated that, in order to take up the 1·5 million new workers per year, at the rate of progress of automation maintained at that time against the resistance of the labour unions, the GNP per capita ought to increase by at least 4·5% p.a. instead of the 3·5% maintained as an average in the previous twenty years.* (It has dropped to a much lower level at the time of writing, in an effort to fight inflation.) But assuming that this increase of 4·5% had been maintained from 1966 until AD 2000 this would have meant a four-and-a-half-fold increase per capita, and a spending power of about $40,000 per family, in 1971 dollars. This, if we take it seriously, would take the US population near to the upper limit of the Post-Industrial Society.

This is what I mean by 'stretching the economy of scarcity

---

* *Technology and the American Economy*, Vol. 1, February 1966. Report of the National Commission on Technology, Automation and Economic Progress.

beyond its natural limits'. Demand will not always outrun supplies. Long before this the stage will be reached when, as David Riesman writes: 'people may discover that a new car every three years instead of every two is quite satisfactory. And once they have two cars, a swimming pool and a boat, and winter and summer vacations, what then?'*

Something will have to give! The consumer society cannot be stretched so far, unless perhaps we invent machines for consumption. If we cannot think of something better, it will come to an end through that *nausea* which is already becoming manifest in the hippies and in the rebellious students.

I believe that there is no need to break with the 'Protestant ethic', with the principle that 'he who does not work, neither shall he eat!' All we have to do is *not* to interpret 'work' as 'production'.

In fact, much that passes nowadays for productive work is sham production. The millions of workers who have become redundant on the production line have been absorbed by the offices. Parkinson's Law was a powerful social factor at the time (1958) when C. Northcote Parkinson wrote his famous book; since that time it has grown to astounding strength. Around 1950 some very able men estimated that ten of the rather slow electronic computers available at that time could do all the computation necessary in the USA; two would suffice for the UK. At the time of writing there are more than 70,000 fast, modern electronic computers in the USA, about 6000 in the UK, most of them in offices, each capable of doing the work of hundreds or thousands of clerks – but the number of office personnel has increased steadily. How much longer can it be before this most wonderful of all labour-saving devices really starts to save labour? Already their computing capacity is far in excess of that of the whole of humanity, doing nothing but computation for 24 hours a day, not even by hand, but with desk machines. Is the business of humanity really so complicated that man must spend all his time doing arithmetic? It would be a bold prophet who would dare to forecast the year of saturation, but at the present rate of

* David Riesman, *Abundance for What?*, Chatto and Windus, London, 1964, p. 175.

increase (still about 25% p.a.) it must be well before the end of the century.

The social consequences of the computer are still largely hidden, but they cannot remain hidden much longer. The analytical minds who devised the computers and their programmes are giving more and more attention to their applications; to the streamlining of services. One cannot quite suppress the suspicion that computer experts are somewhat hampered by their interest in selling more computers, and willing to computerize uneconomical business procedures with far too much paperwork, even adding to it. But sooner or later, in a competitive system, the most economical methods must win. One can imagine these as a combination of 'Marks & Spencer rationalization' with computerization. This great English department-store chain has almost doubled its sales, without computers, with the same personnel, just by cutting out unnecessary paperwork. There is no obstacle to this in the private sector of the Western countries, so long as expansion keeps in step with rationalization, and no staff need be dismissed. This however brings us back to the same dilemma. It will not be possible much longer to boost consumption at the same rate as rationalization and computerization increase the individual efficiency.

The public sector of our economy is likely to defend itself longer against this dilemma than the private one. Every new social service, pension insurance, public assistance, nationalized health service, etc., means the setting up of new offices with thousands of public servants. Every new tax requires a new administration. Moreover there is a possibility of making these new taxes far more complicated than the old ones. When the new English capital gains tax was introduced, the civil servants asked for an extra £100 for the time and effort needed to study the immensely complicated document. In the first year the cost of its administration far exceeded the revenue from this tax. We can expect such practices to grow in strength for some time, because increasing the number of public employees is one of the ways of fighting technological unemployment. I have long regarded Parkinson's Law not so much as a tumour, but as a healthy manifestation of the Protestant ethic. Decent people want to work, because they want to feel socially useful. It would be expecting too much of the state employee to question the justice of the system which gives him bread and employment.

There is, however, one sector of our economy for which efficiency presents no problem because consumption is unlimited, and this is, unfortunately, the armaments industry and the armed forces. There is no need to use up armaments, they become obsolete in a few years and can be sunk in the sea (as happened to much of the surplus equipment left at the end of the war), or converted to scrap iron. This is of course a terrible waste from any Utopian point of view, but unfortunately not from a more realistic one. The obsolete armaments may well have done their duty while they served as *deterrents*. Much as I hate war (like every form of violence) I cannot deny that for a long time we shall not be able to be safe without a minimum of deterrence.

But it is revolting that of all the ways of wasteful spending, it is precisely the most dangerous one, the building up of armaments, which fits best into both the capitalist and the communist systems. For the superproductive Western countries it is a bottomless sink, which never threatens to reach saturation. It keeps many hundred thousands of workers busy in an avant-garde industry, which also employs many of the most inventive technologists. The material needs of man are finite, they do not require immensely complicated machinery for their satisfaction. But when it comes to inventing machines of destruction, pitting one's brain against the best brains on the other side, there is no limit. For a while the urge towards pushing technology to its limit found a harmless outlet in the Space Race, but since the landing on the moon enthusiasm has visibly abated, and at the time of writing the sums spent on it have been sharply reduced.

Armaments also fit only too well into the Soviet system, which has been characterized as a 'total military–industrial complex'. Maintaining a feeling of solidarity among the people of the USSR has not proved to be easier than in the managerial societies of the West. The Soviet leaders have always considered defence their first priority. They have only grudgingly yielded to the popular demand for more consumer goods; 600,000 private motor cars per year will be manufactured in a factory constructed with

Western capital. In a 'petit bourgeois' society, as amply provided with consumer goods as in the Western countries, it would be difficult to maintain the spirit of a 'besieged fortress' surrounded by ruthless, envious enemies. The brilliant anonymous satire *Report from Iron Mountain** alleges that the same is also true for the United States; that only the danger of war can create the social solidarity required for inner peace. The difference is only that what is malicious satire in the USA where the Vietnam war has created nothing but dissension, is still stark reality in the USSR.

It appears that the transition towards a mature society may be equally difficult under the communist and under the capitalist system, though for somewhat different reasons. Both are under the pressure of technological change, with the promise of an easy life for the masses and a difficult life for the administration. In the Soviets it will be delayed by the fear of the rulers, who dread any manifestation of freedom. In the capitalist countries progress is slowed down by the restrictive practices of the workers, who fear unemployment, and of course by the system itself. Capitalism is based on private enterprise, which expects a profit. It is very regrettable that this term has taken on a sinister connotation, as if it meant exploitation. It has now become respectable in some communist countries where the 'New Economic Mechanism' requires every state enterprise to show a profit. But in the advanced Western countries the public or administered sector of the economy is already close to one-half of the whole, and this branch brings at best very meagre profits; for the most part it maintains itself by taxing the other half of the economy. But this is just the part which must be increased in a mature society, as it contains education, public welfare and care of the old. It is not unreasonable to expect that by the end of the century it will have grown from half to about three-quarters of the total economy. Can the private sector be reduced to one-quarter without the whole system collapsing?† Evidently not so long as the other three-quarters continue to be parasitic on this one quarter.

The transition will be difficult, but not impossible. My concern is that it shall not mean the replacement of individual drive by a

---

* *Report from Iron Mountain*, Macdonald, London, 1967.
† See Note 5.

Parkinsonian bureaucracy. Sweden has managed to take a giant step towards the super-welfare state without nationalizing its great industries. Besides, state enterprises need not be stagnant, and their heads need not be sleepy bureaucrats, as has been shown by the examples of Louis Armand in France,* and Enrico Mattei in Italy.† For the great transformation before us we must capture as much as possible of the spirit of early, heroic capitalism, without its cruelties and crudities.

---

* The reorganizer of the French State Railways.
† The super-energetic founder of the Italian State Petrol Trust.

5. TECHNOLOGY AUTONOMOUS

The fear of machines is almost as old as industrial civilization. Oswald Spengler's prophecy that 'Faustian Man will be dragged to death by his own machines' has never been quite forgotten. In a less dramatic form, the 'autonomy' of technology is a danger which is worrying many contemporary thinkers. Will technology remain a faithful servant of human ends, or will it take the bit between its teeth?*

There are two distinct sides to this question. On the one hand, industry based on technology is an essential organ of our civilization; it has a fierce will to survive and for this it must remain profitable. The other side is the equally determined will of creative technologists for producing innovations. These two forces, acting in unison, have indeed created something which seen from the outside appears as 'technology autonomous'.

Technological industry creates the material necessities and luxuries of life, but also plastic bottles, throwaway goods and other sources of solid waste and pollution, and to a great extent it

* See for instance Jacques Ellul, *La Technique*, 1961, translated into English by John Wilkinson as *The Technological Society*, Alfred A. Knopf, New York, 1964. It was the subject of an interesting discussion in the Center for the Study of Democratic Institutions, Santa Barbara, December 1965. But the most formidable critic of technology autonomous is Lewis Mumford, who has recently crowned his great life's work with two volumes of *The Myth of the Machine*, *Technics and Human Development* (1967) and *The Pentagon of Power* (1970), Secker & Warburg, London. I cannot undertake to give a summary of his powerful pleading; it will be better for the reader to take it from him, first-hand. Lewis Mumford has had a great influence on my thinking for more than thirty years. I differ from him in one respect; I am far more suspicious than he of the Nature of Man.

lives on the continual consumption of rapidly wearing articles, as described with great journalistic skill by Vance Packard in his book *The Waste Makers*. It also creates fashions, putting pressure on the consumer to discard motor cars and other 'durables' long before the end of their natural life. I need not enlarge on this. At a conservative estimate, without advertisements, without fashions, without waste, the industrial effort could be reduced by at least a quarter – but what then would the redundant workers do? If they swell the number of the unemployed, they cannot buy even what the remaining three-quarters of industry produces. This is the 'whirling-dervish economy' at its most obvious. We shall not be able to break the vicious circle without a considerable re-direction of manpower, and reforms in financing, such as I will discuss in later chapters.

The other source of the seemingly autonomous drive of technology is of course the self-interest and the mentality of the technologists.* Creative, inventive minds in industry are all the time searching for new products, There is rarely a pre-existing demand for these, because the imagination of the consumers is far behind that of the inventors. In many cases a new product displaces another, as detergents have displaced soap. In others it creates a demand simply by the fact that it appears on the market. Innovations are fuel to the whirling-dervish economy, but in our times this does not work out in all cases. In the most highly developed progressive industries, in which an important innovation must appear every few years, there is a definite tendency for the supply to overshoot the demand.

An obvious example is the aircraft industry. When manned military aircraft became less important, the aircraft industry was able to use a part of its highly skilled manpower for the manufacture of missiles, but not all of it. In Britain as in the United States it became overgrown, but as it could not be allowed to go bankrupt, it turned increasingly towards civilian aircraft, with government support. The jet airliner was thrust on the airlines at a time when they had not yet quite amortized their propeller planes, and for years they went through hard times. Ten years

---

* I wish that there were a new Sinclair Lewis who could expose the human side of technologists as he exposed medical researchers in his *Doctor Arrowsmith*.

later the jumbo jet was thrust on them, which has produced serious losses at the time of writing. It was not as popular with the public as had been expected, and it came at a time when, owing to the recession, the capacity of the airlines overshot the demand. On top of all this came the supersonic airliner. Only the most sanguine optimist could ever expect that the Anglo-French Concorde or the American SST would ever become profitable, yet they had to be developed with taxpayers' money, partly for prestige, but partly to avoid shutting down the most progressive units in the aircraft industry, with their skilled workers and their superlative engineering staff. In 1971 the SST was defeated by a narrow vote in the US Congress. This was historically the first instance of a parliament calling a stop to 'technological progress', and it can be argued that the correct decision was made for not quite the right reasons. It was a majority of conservationists and environmentalists which brought the SST to a halt, not the determination to stop a line of development which was driving *ad absurdum*. Because what will come after the 350–500 seat jumbo and the supersonic plane? The 1000-seat jumbo, and the hypersonic plane? And after that? However much the technologists would hate to admit it, some time the aircraft industry must settle down on a stationary basis, building planes only for replacement, with small improvements, like the motor car industry. It will not have the advantage of the motor industry, which can keep up an exaggerated production by creating fashions, because the customers of the aircraft industry are commercial airlines which must make a profit, and are not as gullible as the general public.

I have separated the innovative drive of the technologists from the whirling-dervish economy of the capitalist system, because it is just as clearly visible in the Soviets.* In the twenties J. M. Keynes thought, like almost everybody else, that no peak achievements of technology could be expected in the communist countries, but only practical, popular techniques, to satisfy primary demands. Exactly the opposite has happened. The

* The capitalist system may not be able to survive without innovations (Note 5), but innovations with much the same priorities can survive without capitalism.

Soviets have produced the first hydrogen bomb, the first ICBM missiles, the first space vehicles and also the first supersonic air liner. One can ascribe the first two achievements to their overwhelming urge for security, but the last two are the result of concentrating their technological elite on prestige projects. On the other hand they still have not produced good harvesters (only inferior copies of American machines), and when it came to the mass production of motor cars they had to turn to Fiat and Renault.

In some matters the rulers of the USSR are better psychologists than democrats. After the war they rebuilt first their factories, then their theatres and human habitations only came third. Friends of mine were invited, only a few years after the war, to Stalingrad, and there to the freshly rebuilt opera house, where they saw a ballet of a magnificence far beyond anything the West could offer. Most of the Russians who came to it in their best clothes had crept out of crumbling, half-destroyed houses, repaired in a rough-and-ready way with wooden props. It was the same psychology which made the USSR put space vehicles before washing machines and motor cars.

The 'Race to the Moon' was also a perfectly logical outcome of the drive of inventors. It is a compulsion for them to look, at every stage of technology, for the next difficult but still feasible objective – and if something *can* be made it *must* be made!* And what is there more difficult and more exciting than a step into space? A moon rocket is a peak performance of technology, it gives work to hundreds of thousands, it realizes an old dream of humanity, and it is also a magnificent phallic symbol. One must admit that the only time when almost the whole population of the world was united not in fear but in hope and pride was the day in 1969 when it watched the first steps on the moon by the crew of Apollo 11, and the second time in 1970 when almost the whole world held its breath over the perilous adventure of Apollo 13. How I wish that the space race were not a dead end – but it is!

I have first-hand knowledge of the compulsion to invent,

* In the words of my fellow-futurist Hasan Ozbekhan, 'every *can* becomes an *ought*'.

because I have lived on it and for it during my long scientific-engineering life. It is wonderful to live with a dream which slowly turns into hardware or into a workable process – even if it is not a practical success in ninety-nine cases out of a hundred. It is not without regrets that I have come to the realization that invention, in the sense of gadgeteering, must come to an end. But the inventive spirit must not perish; it is much too important a part of the creativeness of man. It must now be re-directed, from 'hardware' inventions towards social inventions. I know that many of our inventive spirits will never be able to take this step, but there will be many others who can do it. Technology is not all 'hardware'. In recent decades technologists have moved successfully into more abstract fields, of which the complicated 'software' of modern computers is only a somewhat pedestrian example. There is now developing a great new science of organizing complicated systems towards a goal. Many technologists have become aware of the contrast between the scientific, purposeful organization of engineering projects (such as Polaris, or Apollo) and the haphazard, inadequate processes of society. There exists a potentially powerful army of highly skilled and disciplined thinkers, who are anxious to enter a field for which Olaf Helmer has coined the term 'social technology'.

If only this army of scientists and technologists could be diverted from technology autonomous, and organized for the good of society! Many thousands of them, of the best and most intelligent, are deeply conscious of the fact that we have got our priorities wrong. The avant-garde of technologists are engaged either in war work, or in pyramid-building (the space race), or they are desperately trying to give something 'to the man who has everything'; to the already overloaded consumer society. They are aware that meanwhile the social machinery is creaking and groaning, that it is racked by pollution, by the senseless drive towards Megalopolis, by stagnation, inflation, unemployment, drug traffic and crime! How willing many of the best would be to work instead on law enforcement, city planning, traffic re-organization and the like – if only there were jobs in these lines. (Some of the scientists who have become redundant in the aerospace industries are now driving taxis.)

The reorganization of the creative effort which is now needed exceeds the power of the great philanthropic foundations (though they could do more than they are doing at present); only the State can do it on the right scale. Later on I will try to make suggestions how the State could undertake great reforms without throwing the whole burden on the taxpayer – by *making it pay* for the great corporations to put their creative efforts into the right channels. I am convinced that if the State has the determination, the corporations will be willing to play, rather than be left out of it. Moreover I think that some enlightened leaders of great corporations will be willing to take the lead, if they get support from legislation. My conclusion is that a great work of persuasion will be needed, directed equally at politicians and at corporation presidents, before technology autonomous can be defeated and before the great pool of creative technologists can direct their inventiveness to the problems which really matter.

6.   ON HUMAN NATURE

Il faut de plus grandes vertus pour supporter la bonne fortune que la mauvaise.

La Rochefoucauld

It is fashionable nowadays to say that we still know nothing about Man's nature. Indeed it may be a few hundred years before we have a science of psychology on a level with the 'hard' sciences. I feel inclined to agree with J. B. S. Haldane, who said that about as much thinking will have to go into it as into all the other sciences taken together. But we cannot wait so long in a historical epoch in which Man's condition may change as radically in fifty years as it has in the past five thousand.

Saying that Man in the highly developed countries will soon become a *nouveau riche*, who does not know what to do with himself, is still understating the difficulty of the problem. The *nouveaux riches* of the past soon learned what to do; they took on the social habits of the class into which they had risen by their wealth. This is not a model for a classless, democratic society which has become uniformly rich. At best the masses may model themselves on these exceptional individuals of the leisured classes, for whom life was full of meaning and of interest, though they never had to work hard for their living. Taken as a whole, the class of the rich, the 'undeserving elites' of which I will give a sketch in another chapter, were seldom worthy of imitation.

Psychology has certainly progressed since the time when lunatics were thought to be inhabited by devils, but this would be measuring from a very low level. Freud's exploration of the unconscious ranks with the greatest achievements of the human mind, but his 'meta-psychology', with which he intended to crown his life's work, reducing all human drives to 'Eros' or the 'Pleasure Principle' and to a 'Death Wish', is not likely to survive and does not give much help in practical psychology. Freud never thought that the Age of Leisure could ever be more than a dream; he believed that the economy of scarcity would stay with us for ever. If he had known that all the people could eventually suffer from the same complaints as his rich patients in Vienna, he would probably have been even more pessimistic than he was when he wrote *The Malaise in Civilisation*.

As the greatest of psychologists fails us (and his disciples have not done much better),* I will fall back on a simple homely psychology, based on two observations which most people will be able to check from their own experience, or from their own insight.

I. *Man is wonderful in adversity, weak in comfort, affluence and security.*

II. *Man does not appreciate what he gets without an effort.*

The first of these gives us a warning of the dangers, the second gives a hint how we may perhaps be able to avoid them. I will now illustrate and amplify them.

I. *Man is wonderful in adversity.* Not all of course, but a good many whom in daily life one might take for weaklings. Anybody who saw the rejuvenation of the British people after Dunkirk, when Britain was in mortal danger, can attest to this, but I have even more dramatic examples. Among my friends there are three Hungarian writers who spent years in the prisons and concentration camps of Rákosi's Hungary, between 1949 and 1953.†

---

* I do not deny of course that group-psychologists such as McDougall and Trotter, anthropologists like Ruth Benedict and Margaret Mead and ethologists such as Lorenz and Tinbergen have collected a wealth of important observations. But where is the genius who will synthesize these into a workable theory of social psychology?

† George Faludy, Paul Ignotus, George Páloczi-Horváth. See Faludy, *My Happy Days in Hell*, André Deutsch, London, 1962; Paul Ignotus, *Political Prisoner*, Routledge & Kegan Paul, London, 1961; George Páloczi-Horváth, *The Undefeated*, Secker & Warburg, London, 1959.

Compared with the camp of Recsk, the Siberian concentration camp of Ivan Denisovitch was a holiday camp, because the brutality and sadism of the Hungarian warders left the Russians far behind. All three assert that they have never felt physically better and mentally more alert than when they were fed on mildewed bread, frostbitten potatoes and stone-hard beans – and not much even of these. The powers of resistance which these intellectuals developed is almost unbelievable. One of them, Paul Ignotus, did not notice that he was being tortured when he was shut through a long afternoon into a cabin in which sharp spikes from all sides forced him to stand upright. He thought that it was some unfinished repair work, because he was too intent on thinking out a reply to a question he had received from a fellow intellectual the night before. In Recsk, the intellectuals formed a sort of Academy. They were not of course allowed books of any sort. So they gave up part of their night, after a hard day's work in mud or snow, to discussions and to lectures from memory, in total darkness. One knew something about Byzantium in the 6th century, the other about astronomy; all was food to their thirsty minds. Not one intellectual had a nervous breakdown (though some brutal peasant boys went mad); they came out of their prisons and camps as perfectly balanced individuals.*

The converse. A conversation between a friend of mine, a New York doctor and a lady patient: 'Doctor, I am always so tired!' – 'What makes you so tired?' – 'Getting about.' – 'But you have a Cadillac and a chauffeur!' – 'Yes, but getting in and out is such a fag!' This may read like a bad joke, but I can vouch for its authenticity.

These are of course extreme examples, but I believe that at the present stage of our knowledge of Man's nature we can learn more from extreme examples than from statistics. So long as we have no measure of the state of mind, even statistics become telling only when they refer to extremes. We have no measure of unhappiness, but we can get some idea of it from the suicide figures.

---

* The beneficial effects of semi-starvation deserve attention. In Note 6 I give the testimony of a remarkable witness, the English traveller Mansfield Parkyns whose brilliant description of 'kyef' I have quoted in *Inventing the Future*.

Insecurity produces its neuroses, but so does security. We are talking more of insecurity than ever, but most people may have forgotten the terror of material insecurity which existed not so long ago, when there was no assistance for the unemployed and for the aged. Let me drive this home, again with some extreme examples. Before the First World War, in the USA the insurance premium for the loss of the left arm was less than for the right arm. The insurance companies noticed that there were far more accidents to the left arm than to the right; they equalized the payments and at once the losses became equal. One must conclude that there were unfortunate men, threatened by unrelieved misery once they lost their job, who thrust their arms into the maws of a machine! Equally terrible things happened in the great slump in the thirties, which I remember vividly. The poor, unsuccessful Austrian inventor Marek cut off his foot 'accidentally' with an axe, to get his insurance. A little Hungarian grocer, threatened with bankruptcy, had himself *murdered* (with a hammer!) so that his widow should not remain destitute. (Unsuccessful sacrifices, of course, in both cases.)

And security? Certainly not in all, but in many cases it has the effect on men like the act of which Shakespeare writes:

> The expense of spirit in a waste of shame . . .
> Enjoy'd no sooner than despisèd straight.

By all means let us lift the struggle for life above the level of bare survival. Let us do this out of a sense of the obligation of our rich society to human dignity, but let us not expect that by itself it will stop social unrest.

A phenomenon of the same nature as the contempt of security is the *contempt of freedom*; of the security of thought and speech. The chief hero of the rebellious students and of the radical wing of the communist parties outside the USSR is Mao Tse-Tung, who some years ago announced 'Let a thousand flowers bloom together and a hundred philosophers contend', and then quickly liquidated them when they started to 'contend'.

Was Dostoevsky's Great Inquisitor* right when he said that 'man is tormented by no greater anxiety than to find someone

* In *The Brothers Karamazov*, 1880.

quickly to whom he can hand over that gift of freedom with which that ill-fated creature was born'? Certainly not all of us are anxious to do so, but still far too many who ought to know better. As regards the many, we can add a little correction to the Great Inquisitor's bitter thoughts: 'Turn these stones into bread and mankind will run after Thee like a flock of sheep, grateful and obedient, though for ever trembling lest Thou withdraw Thy hand and deny them Thy bread.' They will take the bread, but they will remain grateful and obedient *only so long* as they are kept trembling.

If men, or at least many men, have this eternal troublemaker in them, how dare I hope for a stationary, rich, secure society? Is the very word 'stationary' not asking for trouble? I will forgo the facile answer, that the troublemakers are only a small minority. We have not yet made the great experiment. The Great War and the Great Slump are still within living memory, and who knows whether the nausea which now affects only a fraction of the young will not spread also to those of more mature age, to the age group which today still remembers the bad old days and is duly grateful for its daily bread and security?

My answer is rather that *individual lives in a stationary society need not be stationary*. At least for the great majority they can be far more adventurous, diversified and challenging than they are in today's 'dynamic' society. This is a subject for a later chapter.

II. *Man does not appreciate what he gets without an effort*. This seems to be such a commonplace that it might appear unnecessary to enlarge on it. Everybody knows spoilt children, spoilt women, perhaps also spoilt men. But our whole technological civilization is running in the direction of getting more with less effort! Why then should it surprise us that schoolchildren and university students want to lessen the effort of learning, and want their representatives to sit on the examining boards? When life has become so easy, why should school be so hard?

Sigmund Freud wrote that the simplest and straightest way of following the Pleasure Principle is *wishing*. Only when wishing fails will man be willing to make a compromise with the Reality Principle, and reach his object by a detour. Now it appears that we can get almost everything by wishing, or by bullying; why not follow these short cuts to pleasure?

I will not dwell on the obvious argument that *everybody* cannot play the spoilt child; somebody still has to do the work. This does not take us very far, because with a highly developed technology all the work of the world could be done by a volunteer minority, who could keep the hedonistic majority in comfortable idleness. Hedonistic minorities, the undeserving elites of the past, have existed for a few generations; a hedonistic majority would, in all probability, hardly survive one generation.

There also exists, however, a contrary tendency in human nature which does not only ask for an effort; it asks for *sacrifices*. This is a specifically human trait; animals are free from it. Right at the beginnings of *homo sapiens*, in the Pyrenean caves we find fearful evidence of this human madness; the imprints of mutilated hands, with fingers missing. Were the victims dragged by force to the chopping block, or were they volunteers?* I am inclined to think that they were volunteers, who believed in the necessity of a sacrifice in an epoch when the dark, diffuse religion of the time was a hundred per cent fear, even if some forceful persuasion had to be exerted at the last moment. I take the mutilated hands to be the precursors of the self-mutilating zealots of later religions, rather than of the victims of the terrible human sacrifices of the Mayas and Aztecs. But who knows whether the virgin whose heart was torn out by the Aztec priest did not also believe in the necessity of the sacrifice? However this may be, there was in *homo sapiens* from the beginning a deep feeling of guilt which has prevented him from enjoying the simple happiness of animals, and which, short of a mutation, will prevent him from following the Pleasure Principle along the straight path, except for short intervals.

I can see no evidence that this basic feeling of guilt can be eradicated, in those who have it, by methods known to us. Not even by psychoanalysis. I once asked one of the doyens of psychoanalysis: 'You must have known just about all the psycho-

* There is a most convincing reconstruction of such a mutilation in William Golding's novel, *The Inheritors* (Faber, London, 1958), which suggests that it was voluntary.

analysts, from Freud and Ferenczi onwards. Have you ever known a healthy and happy psychoanalyst?' He replied: 'When I meet a healthy and happy psychoanalyst, I will send you a cable.'

Arthur Koestler argues that this belief in human sacrifices, even in self-sacrifice, is a built-in evolutionary error in Man, which is likely to lead him to destruction, unless we can produce the equivalent of a mutation by drugs not yet discovered.* He may well be right: collective madnesses of the type of religious wars may yet recur. But these mental epidemics do not occur by 'spontaneous combustion', they require leaders, organizations, and a watchful society ought to be able to stifle the chain-reaction at an early stage. What is likely to remain, the *individual* will to solidarity and sacrifice, can then be canalized into constructive channels, as all successful civilizations have done in their heyday. How to do this, in the absence of the pressure of economic necessity, is one of the chief problems this book discusses.

---

* Arthur Koestler, *The Ghost in the Machine*, Hutchinson, London, 1967. Pacifying drugs, such as *Diazopan*, are known which turn the wickedest boss-monkey into a pacificist, but this does not satisfy Koestler, because he thinks that monkeys are free from the specifically human urge for identification and self-sacrifice.

7. THE MORAL ACHIEVEMENTS OF SCIENCE

Can we find in history a proof of the moral progress of mankind? The pessimist can say: 'Genghis Khan is said to have erected a pyramid of human eyes. Only pyramids of human spectacles have been found in the Nazi extermination camps. Is this moral progress?' But the optimist can reply: 'In the great Irish potato famine of 1847–49, at least a million Irish men, women and children starved to death while England turned its back on them and gave only quite insufficient aid. A hundred years later, in 1946, in the great rice famine in Bengal, the British Government forbade all rice exports from India, though the people of England would have welcomed the rice after the scarcity of the war years. This *is* moral progress.' The pessimist is right in warning us of the possibility of terrible relapses, but I am on the side of the optimist. There is a trend in the history of morals towards the better, and I believe that it will continue. The teachings of the great founders of religions and of moralists have not permanently prevailed against the dark sides of human nature, but now they have a powerful ally in science.

It is a fashionable stupidity of our time to reproach science for not having an ethical content, and therefore to be equally capable of being used for good or for evil. Indeed, science is ethically neutral, but even neutrality is better than a bias towards evil. It was this neutrality which enabled science to achieve great moral improvements in human society, first of all by *driving out superstitions*.

Man differs from animals in that he has a reasoning mind, and this mind has a sinister bias. It cannot tolerate a vacuum, it finds an explanation for everything, and in the pre-scientific mind the explanations and the remedies were mostly cruel and sadistic. I heard an unforgettable example of this, when in 1951, on a visit to the Research Laboratory of the General Electric Company I heard on the same day of the pre-scientific and the scientific methods of rain-making. In the evening, one of the Great Old Men, William D. Coolidge,* gave a talk on his visit to the Maya Peninsula, and described the Maya method of making rain. The Maya (or Aztec) priest broke the breasts of virgins with a stone axe, tore out the palpitating heart, and threw the corpse into the sacred pond. Thousands of these mutilated skeletons of young girls were found in these ponds. A little earlier, another Great Old Man, Irving Langmuir,† had explained to me his scientific method of rain-making, by injecting silver iodide crystals into saturated clouds. This may not be a very safe method either, but I believe that it constitutes some progress over that of the Mayas and Aztecs.‡

The civilization of the Mayas and Aztecs may have been a particularly sick one, but when the Christian Spaniards broke into Mexico and Peru they did not behave like the representatives of a higher and more humane civilization. It was the epoch of the Inquisition, when the Spanish towns were often reeking with the stench of burned human flesh. And it was just at the beginning of the two terrible centuries of the Witch Hunt. Here again, in Christian Europe, we find the sinister reasoning of the pre-scientific mind. 'The cow gives no milk, so the old witch next door must have bewitched her.' I wonder, were not more old women put to painful death in Christian Europe than virgins in Mexico?

Driving out superstitions was the first moral achievement of science. It is still far from complete, because according to an estimate of the physicist Edward U. Condon, there are at present

* Inventor of the malleable tungsten filament and of the modern X-ray tube.

† One of the greatest of applied scientists. Inventor of the gas-filled incandescent lamp and of the hard-vacuum electron valve.

‡ An even more horrifying example was the pre-scientific 'technique' of tempering Toledo steel daggers in the bowels of slaves. The useless tortures to which the ignorant physicians of the past subjected their unfortunate patients belong to the same chapter.

in the USA about 10,000 people gainfully employed in astrology, and only 2000 in astronomy. Connecting human fate with the position of the planets at the hour of birth is of course an egregious stupidity, but at least it is not sadistic. Still, I find it a disturbing thought that there are so many people among us with pre-scientific minds. If they swallow this nonsense, they may be ready to accept others, more harmful.

The second great moral achievement of science was that *it made physical pain unnecessary.* So long as there was no better pain-killer than brandy, the surgeon had to be a sadist himself. Usually the patient who had to have a limb amputated was made dead drunk, but the surgeon too had a good swig of some strong drink. Anaesthesia in surgical operations was introduced comparatively late (by W. T. G. Morton in the USA in 1846, by J. Y. Simpson in Britain in 1847), but a powerful painkiller, morphine, was isolated from opium in 1806 by the German apothecary F. W. A. Sertürner, who deserves to be remembered as one of the great moral improvers of mankind. So long as pain was unavoidable, the common people delighted not only in public tooth-pulling by the barber at the fairs, but also in public executions. Not many people nowadays could stand the sight of the tumbril moving slowly through the streets of a town, with the delinquent tied to a stake, and the executioner with the brazier next to him digging the red-hot poker into the screaming wretch. In our time millions of innocent people have been put to death in extermination camps, but the guards were carefully selected brutes; no dictator has dared to make a public spectacle of it. Remember also that Cruelty is conspicuously missing from the Seven Deadly Sins. If now we abhor it even more than the others, this is, I believe, due in great part to the fact that physical pain is no longer an unavoidable component of human life.

Modern science has also recently defeated a great source of mental anguish. Nature does not seem to care much about men reaching a happy post-maturity – they lose their eyesight and their teeth. But Nature is much more cruel to women, many of whom never get over the hormonal deficiency which starts with the climacteric. When the woman is past child-bearing age, Nature casts her away, like a squeezed-out lemon. The 'change of

life' has caused untold suffering to women, their husbands and
their families. The great biochemists who have isolated and
synthesized the sex hormones have made an immeasurable
addition to human happiness. Almost everybody, men and
women, can now expect to have a happy period of post-maturity,
which in the past was given only to those with exceptionally
lucky constitutions.

Most of our contemporary intellectuals, in their impatience
with the imperfections of our society, tend to forget these things.
Let me remind them of the moral progress which they have made
themselves, as compared to the thinkers of a hundred years ago, not
by any merit of their own, but by the progress of science and
technology. Here is a quotation from David Ricardo, who
according to the report of all his contemporaries was an exceptionally mild and benevolent man:

'It is a truth which admits not a doubt, that the comforts and
well-being of the poor cannot be permanently secured without
some regard on their part, or some effort on the part of the
legislature, to regulate the increase of their numbers and to
render less frequent among them early and improvident marriages.
The operation of the system of Poor Laws has been directly
contrary to this.'*

And this is a quotation from John Stuart Mill:

'. . . most persons who can afford it pay their domestic servants
higher wages than would purchase the labour of persons fully as
competent to the work required. They do this, not merely from
ostentation, but also for more reasonable motives; either because
they desire that those they employ should serve them cheerfully,
and be anxious to remain in their service . . . or because they
dislike to have near their persons and continually in their sight
people with the appearance and habits which are the usual
accompaniments of mean remuneration. . . . But they can never
raise the average wages of labour beyond the ratio of population
to capital. By giving more to each person employed, they limit
the power of giving employment to numbers, and however

* *The Works and Correspondence of David Ricardo*, edited by Piero Sraffa and
M. H. Dobb, Cambridge, 1951. Chapter V, 'On Wages', pp. 106–7. First
Edition 1817.

excellent their moral effort, they do little good economically, unless the pauperism of those who are shut out leads indirectly to a readjustment by means of an increased restraint on population.'*

These warnings against 'pampering the poor' by the poor laws or by higher remuneration strike us as barbaric. But if David Ricardo was a mild, kind man, John Stuart Mill can be characterized as angelic, and both were influenced by Thomas Robert Malthus, who was equally angelic. They just could not see any way for improving the situation of the poor other than by reducing their numbers, which meant sexual restraint and late marriages. That the cake could grow faster than the number of 'the poor' was as far from their minds as The Pill. Certainly, we still have to utter warnings against overpopulation, but we do not address them to 'the poor' but to everybody. We expect the poorer brackets only to take on the habits of the middle classes, which in J. S. Mill's time would have meant six to ten children per family. And we do not expect them to remain poor at all.

This is the moral progress of sociologists in a hundred-odd years in the highly industrialized, rich countries. But even when we address ourselves to the underdeveloped countries, whose level of material prosperity is still rather below that of England a hundred years ago, we do not express pious hopes that 'their pauperism will lead to increased restraint on population', we do not preach at them, but offer them modern technology and The Pill – the medicine which we have taken ourselves, and which we are taking in increased doses.

Driving out superstitions, eliminating physical pain, relieving hormonal weaknesses, defeating poverty, these are not the last words of science. But the next steps will not be easy, because to a considerable extent these will have to fight the evil effects of science. Morphine has relieved pain, and even when it was taken as a drug, it was not much worse than opium, with which Chinese civilization was able to co-exist for 2000 years. But when chemists derived heroin from it, they produced the killer drug which is now a cancer of American civilization and one of the

* John Stuart Mill, *Principles of Political Economy* (first published 1848), Longmans, Green & Co., London, 1920, p. 404 (end of Chapter XIV).

mainsprings of its growing criminality. I am convinced that with sufficient determination by making it a *project*, like Polaris or Apollo, the drug traffic could be exterminated in a year or two. But this could not suppress the *causes* which now lead to heroin addiction. Suppressing the drug traffic could be a political-military-engineering action, but suppressing the causes also demands change in the psychology of the unfortunates who have now become victims of heroin. These causes go to the very roots of human nature, but I am confident that if some of the best brains of the next generations concentrate on the problem, it too can be defeated. But it will require an immeasurably greater amount of thought than was needed for converting morphine into heroin.

8. UNDESERVING ELITES OF THE PAST

Can people survive in a style of life in which they have no material worries from the cradle to the grave, without work and without making themselves socially useful, and yet without falling into boredom and having to reach for drinks or drugs? Apparently there are some people who can, in a certain social atmosphere. Barbara Tuchman writes that around the turn of the century there were in England about a quarter of a million persons with no specific occupations, idlers, *not* unemployed.★ I find this quite credible: among my friends in London, there are two hard-working elderly gentlemen whose Victorian fathers never did a stroke of work in all their lives. They just got up late, went to the barber, then to the club, playing billiards in the afternoon, cards in the evening. They were quite happy letting other people do the work for them while they lived on their family fortunes.

This type, if it still exists at all, is now becoming very rare, and not only because family fortunes in England are being swallowed up by death duties. An atmosphere has developed in which the idler feels guilty. In the United States this social climate was established long ago. William James records that when he went to school, in the middle of the 19th century, he was ashamed to confess to his schoolmates that his valetudinarian and philosophically inclined father Henry was not in some line of 'business'.

I have attempted thumbnail sketches of four 'undeserving

★ Barbara W. Tuchman, *The Proud Tower*, Macmillan, London-New York, 1966.

elites' – Imperial Rome, Versailles at the time of the Sun King, the Italian and the English aristocracies. By calling them 'undeserving' I do not mean to imply that they did not have some highly deserving members; in the case of the English aristocracy I even think that they have done their country a great service. I mean only that they lived on the work of other people. not by their own wits, but by the accident of birth. I would contrast them with the Church, which on the whole was a meritocracy. If we are planning for an affluent Post-industrial Society we can learn far more from the Church than from these hereditary elites.

Some of the examples below show that hedonism leads to sterility, boredom and decadence, others show that an undeserving elite can survive, at least for a long time – just because it takes pride in being a closed society. There is not much hope to be gathered from this for a uniformly wealthy society: the simple fact is that distinction cannot be distributed democratically!

IMPERIAL ROME

Ancient Rome, in the first three centuries after Christ, is the greatest historical experiment in leisure, and the most frightening. During the apogee of the Empire the city of Rome had a population of between $1\frac{1}{2}$ and 2 million.* Those who never worked may have numbered perhaps half a million, but the rest did not work hard either by our standards. The Roman working day was seven hours in summer and six in winter, but there were not many working days. At the time of Augustus there were 93 public holidays when the Romans were entertained at the expense of the State, to which must be added 45 *feriae publicae* such as the Lupercalia-Saturnalia, a total of 138. By the time of Claudius the number had grown to 159, while the Calendar of Philocalus, written in AD 354, records 175 days of games out of 200 public holidays – more than one for each working day.

* Some modern authors disbelieve this figure and doubt whether it ever exceeded half a million. I cannot believe that the Circus Maximus and the theatres could have taken a full half of the population – slaves and all!

According to Jerome Carcopino,* 150,000 paupers were fed at State expense by Annona Augusta, the Divinity of Imperial Supplies, who had a temple in Ostia, the principal port of Rome. They received not only their measure of flour and oil but, like the other free Romans, their obulus for the bath and their entrance badge for the games. Almost all the other free Romans were the *clientes* of somebody, and received money or food (*sportula*) from their patrons, to whom they had to pay daily or at least frequent *obsequia*.

The number of idlers can be estimated from the fact that the Circus Maximus had 250,000 seats, and three theatres together had another 30,000. The Colosseum, begun under Vespasian (AD 69–79) held about 50,000. It is a marvel of architectural art and ingenuity but history did justice to their builders by not preserving their names. They were indeed spiritual brothers to the German engineers who constructed the 'economical' incinerators for the Nazi extermination camps.

The shows in the theatres are the eternal shame of Imperial Rome, and a sad proof of the corruptibility of human nature. Boredom could not be tolerated! 'A people that yawns is ripe for a revolution,' writes Carcopino. 'Finally the emperors, deliberately pandering to the murderous lust of the crowds, found in gladiatorial games the most sinister of the instruments of power.' 5000 beasts were killed in one day of the *munera* with which Titus inaugurated the Colosseum in AD 80. Domitian (AD 81–96) initiated another step in depravity. In the popular play on the life and death of the brigand Laureolus he 'allowed the play to end with a scene in which a criminal condemned under the common law was substituted for the actor and put to death with tortures in which there was nothing imaginary'. And Martial sang the praise of the prince who made these things possible! It appears, though, that Domitian was somewhat half-hearted about cruelty, because in AD 86 he tried to introduce the

* Jerome Carcopino, *Daily Life in Ancient Rome*, first in French, many translations, first US edition New Haven Univ. Press, 1940. A matchlessly brilliant piece of history. Deserves to be better known than Sienkiewicz's *Quo Vadis*, which accuses the Romans of almost the only crime which they did *not* commit: the persecution of the Christians under Nero.

Agon Capitolinus, games in the Greek style, without bloodshed, but these did not catch on. Gladiatorial games were not suppressed in the West until AD 404 under Honorius.

Not the least repulsive feature of Imperial Rome was its complete intellectual sterility. The great Latin poets, Horace, Ovid, Virgil, were long dead. The saltless epigrams and satires of Martial and Juvenal would not be nowadays accepted even in provincial journals – except perhaps in the gossip column. A complete vacuum of creativity, just at the epoch at which the Romans were the masters of the Earth. No wonder Imperial Rome died – the surprising fact is that it died so slowly.

VERSAILLES UNDER THE SUN KING

At the time when France was the most populous country in Europe, with a total of about 15 million souls, it had an aristocracy numbering about 100,000. Some of these were feudal princes, lording it over whole provinces. From Louis XI on (1461–83), the history of France is blood-red with the cruel wars between the monarch and the feudal lords, who were only half subdued in the middle of the 17th century. When in 1661 Louis XIV, to all accounts a very able man, took the reins firmly in his hands, he had a better idea than besieging their fortified mansions one by one. He decided to create a court of such unheard-of magnificence that the most powerful representatives of the proud French nobility would gather around it voluntarily. When the Palace of Versailles took shape (the central part was finished in 1678; the whole is said to have cost a thousand million francs) the highest nobility competed for posts in the royal household. Louis XIV had an instinctive understanding of the importance of ritual, or perhaps he followed oriental examples; he instituted a rigid and elaborate etiquette, and made the nobles its slaves. To hold the candle while the King was undressing was a most valued distinction. The *levée* took three hours. The services of 498 persons were used to provide the King with a meal. Three persons and seven to eight minutes were required to serve him with a glass of wine or water at dinner. (Incidentally, there was not even a vestige of comfort in all this pomp and circumstance. The kitchen was a good quarter mile from the dining-room, and gold plates were either too hot or too cold.)

Alas, the strict etiquette and the pomp could make the nobles forget that they could have been lords in their own chateaux while they inhabited an attic in the palace, but it could not defeat boredom. Jacques Levron writes: 'As a relief to the heavy tedium which from the beginnings of the century weighed upon Versailles, receptions, the visits of illustrious persons, kings, princes or receptions of ambassadors, and births and deaths gave some element of the unexpected to the established routine.... Everyone was bored, and as it was vital to maintain conversation, people became excited over the most futile subjects. Madame de Maintenon's cold, or the fact that the King had been bled, led to endless commentary.'*

Gondolas on the canals, with gondoliers brought from Venice, with singers as night entertainment, were perhaps sufficient for dispelling the tedium for one night. But the boredom, which must have been acute at the beginning, must have become endemic, and bearable to some extent, like syphilis in a country where everybody has it. Even after the death of the Sun King, the nobles with few exceptions did not return to their estates. The courtiers remained tied to their comatose state, while pretending to enjoy themselves with such inanities as pastoral scenes and plays. By the time of the French Revolution, the nobility was approaching the state of the *eloi* in H. G. Wells' *The Time Machine*; ready if not to be eaten, at least to be guillotined.

It was as undeserving an elite as ever existed. The real elite of France, the Huguenots, the most serious, industry-minded part of the population, who would almost certainly have made France the richest and strongest industrial country in Europe, and prevented the revolution, had been expelled long ago. By the revocation of the Edict of Nantes (1685), Louis XIV had unwittingly prepared the ruin of his house, just at the time when Versailles was blooming out in its morning glory.

In all fairness, one must bear in mind that, although Imperial

* Jacques Levron, *Daily Life at Versailles in the 17th and 18th Centuries,* Macmillan, New York, 1968.

Rome and Versailles are frightening examples of human corrupt-ibility, there was the mitigating circumstance that both were corrupted *from above*. This may to some extent excuse the corrupted 'elites', but it provides a lesson for all time: how dangerous may be the expedients for *appeasement* applied by short-sighted rulers.

THE ITALIAN ARISTOCRACY

The great Italian aristocratic families have shown a remarkable power of survival. There are still Orsinis, Colonnas, Barberinis, della Roveres, Sforzas, Viscontis, and many of them are still living in their ancient palaces. All these princely dynasties were founded by outstandingly energetic men. Almost every family history is worthy of a novel, but seldom an edifying one.

It is a curious fact that in seven centuries of brilliant Italian achievements in the arts and sciences we find hardly one aristo-cratic name among the great men. But as soon as the aristocracy was officially abolished by the Republic (which incidentally resulted in a doubling of the number of titled persons), two first-class talents emerged; the Princes Giuseppe di Lampedusa and Luchino Visconti.

The Italian aristocracy in the 19th century, a period in which they were no longer in danger of being exterminated by their neighbours and rivals, or of being exiled by local republican revolutions, is a rather interesting one, because it is a prime example of a 'Society' which lives by 'inviting or not inviting one another' (Ortega y Gasset). In other words, by being a *closed* elite, or even simpler by snobbery. A gifted plebeian snob, Gabriele d'Annunzio, has left credible descriptions of the life of the Roman aristocratic society in the late 19th century.* Somehow they managed to lead a life which consisted of daily parties where they met the same people again and again, depositing their visiting cards on them next morning, meeting them again on horseback or in carrozzas, with an added mixture of duels, horse races, gambling, flirtation and seduction, without falling into excessive boredom,

* In most of his novels, but particularly in *Il Piacere* (Pleasure), 1889.

without excessive drinks or drugs. (Their recent successors, the motley international crowd of the *Dolce Vita*, were not so lucky.) Of course one must take into account that this elaborate game was played out in splendid palaces, with the unique beauty of erstwhile Rome as a backdrop, and that making conversation with the same people (who had little time or inclination to read) was made easy by the wonderful Italian fluency, but yet one must wonder at their stamina. Was it a selection of people adapted by breeding to continuous silken dalliance? I would rather think that they not only survived but enjoyed an unnaturally hedonistic style of life simply by taking pride in the fact that so few people were admitted to it.

THE ENGLISH ARISTOCRACY

George Orwell, one of the most sincere of socialists, wrote that 'our aristocracy is the envy of the world', and he was substantially right. How is it that the English aristocracy has escaped the fate of its French and Russian counterparts, and has survived to the present time when it is being quietly killed by taxes and death duties? We must certainly class it with the 'undeserving' elites, because it was founded partly by the Norman knights who came over with William the Conqueror, and in greater part by those whom Henry VIII rewarded with the estates of the rebels and of the expropriated clergy. There is no reason to consider them as a meritocracy by the 18th century or after it. One may perhaps suppose that there was some eugenic selection at work, because the aristocrats could select their wives from among the most beautiful women, not only of their own class but also of the gentry.* Indeed a glance at them on any occasion when they are assembled in numbers will prove that they are physically not a random sample of the population, but there is no need to suppose

* Francis Galton has spotted a certain 'anti-eugenic' tendency. The aristocrats who were keen on enlarging their estates often married the only daughters of landed families, that is to say they made their selection among the less fertile, thereby making the extinction of their own line more probable. But this would affect only the number, not the quality, of the survivors.

that they are an intellectual elite. In six centuries they have produced six great talents – Chaucer, Boyle, Cavendish, Shelley, Churchill and Bertrand Russell – which is about the number which one could expect from their proportion, and rather less if one considers their opportunities. Yet, this aristocracy has displayed a certain political wisdom, which preserved it to this day, and it has done great services to its country.

They certainly had one advantage over the French aristocracy. There never was a court in England comparable to Versailles which could have corrupted them. They stayed on their estates, or in their great town houses, and went to the court only for short visits, if at all. On the other hand, they did not display any greater love for the common people than did the French. The 'enclosures', which started in the late Middle Ages and went on into the 18th century, displaced hundreds of thousands of unfortunate peasants, who became vagabonds. 'Sheep who used to eat grass now eat men,' wrote Thomas More, at the time when farms were destroyed to make more grazing land for the sheep whose wool was sent to Flanders, to be exchanged for gold and luxuries. Nor was there, even much later, any *camaraderie* between officers and men in the British Army. Wellington's officers fought gallantly beside the men in the front ranks, but they left the care of their troops to their sergeants. As late as the 19th century, lusty peasant boys who poached a rabbit were mercilessly transported to penal colonies.

Yet there was no peasant revolt in England after Wat Tyler, in 1381. The wave of the terrible peasant wars which shook many countries on the Continent in the 16th century never reached the English shores. The only anti-aristocratic revolution in England, the Cromwellian, was a comparatively mild affair. Marxist writers class it as a 'bourgeois' revolution, and there is of course some truth in this, but it leaves out the immensely strong religious emotions of those times. It is indeed somewhat difficult for the modern reader to put himself into the mind of people to whom 'salvation or damnation' was as important as 'bread or starvation'.*
Anyway, the greater part of the aristocracy survived the Republic

* Even the 'Levellers', the left wing of the Roundheads, whom one can well call early socialists, argued with religious arguments. See Joseph Needham,

without much trouble. Only a part of the catholic aristocracy had to go into temporary exile.

Perhaps a revolt would yet have occurred in the late 18th century, had it not been for two things. One was the good sense of the English aristocracy which inclined them, unlike the French, not to oppose the rising bourgeoisie, but rather to help them with capital, and to make political alliances with them. The other was, as is often suggested, the providential appearance of John Wesley (1703–91) on the English scene. This great preacher and organizer preached 'daily growth in holiness, and victory over sin' to the poor people of England. Did the aristocrats understand what a powerful ally they had in him for pacifying the poor and making them forget their grievances? Certainly not all, as may be judged from a letter written by the Duchess of Buckingham in 1741 to Lady Huntingdon:

'I thank your ladyship for the information concerning the Methodist preachers; their doctrines are most repulsive, and strongly tinctured with impertinence and disrespect towards their superiors, in perpetually endeavouring to level all ranks and do away with distinctions. It is monstrous to be told that you have a heart as sinful as the common wretches that crawl on the earth.'*

This is the perfect English counterpart to Marie Antoinette's alleged (probably apocryphal) saying 'Why do they not eat grass?',† but it did not propagate from mouth to mouth. If there was to be no English guillotine, this was hardly the fault of such titled ladies as the Duchess of Buckingham!

The English aristocracy was unique also in another respect.

'Laud, the Levellers and the Virtuosi', in *Time the Refreshing River*, Unwin Brothers, 1943.

Is the horrifying civil war which at the time of writing is going on in Northern Ireland a religious war? I would rather call it a *derivative* religious war. The Catholics and the Protestants do not want to convert each other; the Catholics are fighting against discrimination which they had to suffer because of their religion.

* M. Dorothy George, *England in Johnson's Day*, Harcourt, Brace & Co., New York, 1928.

† Another version is 'Let them eat cakes (*brioches*)', probably equally apocryphal.

They *did* go to excesses in hard drinking, and William Pitt drank himself to death, yet he served his country wonderfully well in one of its darkest hours. He was not the only great English statesman to drink hard. There is an element of luck in the history of England which made it almost always produce the right man at the right time, and I do not think that the example of the English elite is one which could serve as a model in all of its features. Except one, to which we will return later, its instinctive recognition of the importance of *hardship*, exemplified in the great English Public Schools.

9.　THE DIVERSITY OF MAN

Until fairly recently in human history only a minority had the chance to develop their full personality. The others were cast, more or less forcibly, into roles as slaves, serfs, factory workers. The democracy of ancient Athens was based, roughly, on 20,000 free men and 200,000 slaves. The Greeks justified this egregious injustice by the sophism that the slave had proved to be no better than a slave by not committing suicide. Christianity granted an immortal soul to the slave, but did not do much more about him. Only the machine age made it possible to raise the ideal of a democracy with perfect social justice, in which every man had a chance of developing his full personality, and is treated according to his merits. 'Merit' of course meant social usefulness. The technological age has taken us a step further in the hierarchy of lofty ideals. 'To each according to his needs', like the *fraternité* of the French Revolution, used to be nothing but an empty slogan. In the age of affluence, or even of abundance, we can and must take it seriously.

The needs of people must be satisfied, almost regardless of their social merit, for two entirely different reasons. One is the ethical postulate that nobody shall suffer unjust hardship. The other is the consideration of stability; a society in which many people are unhappy cannot be stable. These are two 'complementary' views, which happily do not conflict too much with one another. The ethical argument is emotionally the more appealing, but in fairness one must point out that it is not uncontested.

Elevating humanity to a higher degree of civilization will not be possible without elevating it to a higher *moral* level. So far, what is called in the English-speaking countries the 'Protestant ethic' has been sufficient as a moral mainstay; it will not be sufficient in the future. It needed only a minimum of human decency to recognize that the 'toiling masses', who by producing goods maintained the whole of the society, deserved social justice. But when, by the progress of technology, the toiling masses are no longer needed, justice will have to find other foundations than in the times of economic scarcity. We have come a long way since Herbert Spencer loudly protested against 'pampering the poor' from the rates paid by the affluent. Assistance not only to the unemployed, but also to the unemployable, is now paid in all civilized countries, but only to an extent which keeps them well below the poverty level. When, as can be expected, their number increases and their standard of living is raised to a decent level, we can expect not only protestations but strong resistance from people who by old-fashioned standards consider themselves thoroughly ethical.

This had to be said, but having said it, I will discard the ethical argument and consider the problem of social justice entirely from the point of stability. How can we make a reasonable compromise between the needs and wishes of individuals, and the requirements of a highly developed technological society?

If we are to tackle this problem rationally, we must first of all take account of the tremendous diversity of human characters. It is perfectly useless to talk of 'man' (or 'woman') or of 'average man'. Men share only the primary needs of food, shelter and clothing, and there are enormous differences even in these elementary appetites once a very low minimum is satisfied. When it comes to 'higher' interests, it is hard to believe that we are one species. Bertrand Russell as an adolescent was very unhappy and kept from suicide only by the desire to learn more mathematics. Others, far more numerous, could be driven near to suicide if they were forced to learn mathematics.

Human individuals are so vastly diverse, that it would be hopeless to construct a scheme of classification which could do justice to every one of them. No society, however perfect, can provide a perfect fit for all individuals. It can attempt a compromise with their aspirations, but it cannot avoid *using* them as social building blocks. The classification which I have attempted may be, at least for a start, sufficient for the social engineer who wants to know his material.*

THE INTELLIGENCE QUOTIENT

Intelligence, the ability for problem solving, is the first component of the human character which has found a satisfactory quantitative measure. Though it is a matter of almost daily discussion in newspapers and magazines, it may not be superfluous to give first a brief outline of the 'intelligence quotient' or 'IQ'. Alfred Binet, starting in 1896, was the first to devise batteries of test problems, suitable for school children of 6 to 14 years. The 'mental age' was the battery in which the child reached the *median* of school children of that age, that is to say if he scored as well as half of them. The originator of what we nowadays call IQ was Lewis Terman of Stanford. Starting from Binet's conception, in 1916, he gradually simplified the method, until in 1937 he stabilized the procedure as follows: 'Take a group of people, for instance an age group of school children. Give them a battery of test problems of increasing difficulty, so devised that two-thirds to three-quarters of them can solve about half of the problems, and do not make the difficulties near the top increase too steeply. Give these test problems marks, add up the marks for each person, and *rank* them according to the marks. Arrange your ranked population in percentiles (i.e. divide them up into those which are 1, 2 . . . per cent above the bottom). Allot to these IQs according to a certain standard table whose graphical representation is shown in Fig. 1.' This is a Gaussian normal probability curve, with a standard deviation of 16·14%. (This curious figure is a historical relic, it is now often replaced by 16 or 15.)

* I am not learned enough to give even a thumbnail sketch of the history of characterology, or of its present status. Correspondence with a distinguished expert on the 'measurement of man', H. L. Eysenck, has encouraged me to believe that the line which I am taking; the 'IQ-EQ diagram' and its further extension has some new features.

Two important comments must be made about the IQ. One is that it does not signify anything absolute, it is merely the standing, as regards intelligence, of the individual in the group in which he was tested. Statements such as 'if it were possible to raise the IQ of the population by 5 points . . .' are nonsensical, unless they read: 'raising (by some influence), the intelligence

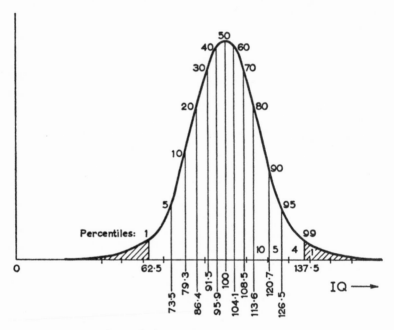

FIGURE I   *The standard IQ scale. Every division contains* 10% *of the population except the shaded divisions, which contain* 1% *each, and the ones next to them, which contain* 4% *and* 5%.

of the individuals in the population so that re-tested *one by one* in the same *old* population their IQ would be higher by 5 points'. One can, possibly, raise the intelligence of a whole population, but not its IQ; it is represented always by the same normal probability curve, with the median at 100. (If one does not understand this, one may as well deplore the fact that 'half of the population has not even average intelligence'.) Another, somewhat more sophisticated, but even less excusable, error is the familiar statement, that 'if it were possible to raise the average IQ of the population by 10 points, the number of high-class talents above an IQ of 130 would increase from 2·4% to 9·4%'. This is nonsense, even if one reformulates it by 're-testing in the old population'. There exists no reason whatever why the histogram thus obtained should be the normal probability curve, shifted without deformation.

On the other hand it makes sense to take out of a total population a *subset* characterized by some distinctive property such as 'one of five or more siblings' or 'only child', plot its histogram, and look at its differences against the normal curve. Such a subset can have a median or average different from 100, and it need not be (and hardly ever will be) a normal probability curve. This in fact is the main method in searching for the factors which determine intelligence.

The other comment is that the compact character of the standard IQ curve, in which 99·7% of the population fall into the apparently narrow limits of 55 and 145, can easily conceal to the uninitiated the enormous scale which it covers. 55 means an imbecile, 145 a man or woman in the top 0·25% of their group. This span covers about three grades of intelligence, which one can rightly say are qualitatively different. The IQ of 145 can solve problems *on inspection*, which one can only just explain to those with 110, but which they are unable to solve, however long they take over it, and so forth, from 110 to 80, from 80 to 55. IQ tests for geniuses have not yet been constructed, because one cannot expect the IQ-specialists to be geniuses, but one must suspect that the scale continues upwards to giddy heights of ability. Most of those who have known the mathematician John von Neumann have felt as slow and stupid in his presence as the dunce with the top of the form.

The IQ scale under-emphasizes rather than over-emphasizes the inequality of men, but this has not saved it from attacks. Research into the sources of intelligence has become political dynamite in the United States. Arthur R. Jensen's scholarly investigation on the influence of hereditary and environmental factors on intelligence and scholastic achievement[*] has provoked

* Arthur R. Jensen, 'How much can we boost IQ and scholastic achievement?', *Harvard Educational Review*, Vol. 39, No. 1, Winter 1969.

great unease and resentment in intellectual circles because he dared to marshal the facts (by no means all new or unknown) regarding the lower IQ of the American Negro, and to dispute the arguments of those who wanted to explain this by 'environmental deprivation'. According to Jensen, and many other researchers, there can be no doubt about environmental influences, but they are far less important than the genetic factors. He protests against those who consider research on these matters untimely or premature. 'To rule out of court, so to speak, any reasonable hypothesis on purely ideological grounds is to argue that static ignorance is preferable to reality.' After proving from statistical material that the dysgenic differential breeding of the socially lowest and least intelligent part of the Negroes threatens to make the problem even worse in future, he writes, in perhaps his most important conclusion: 'The possible consequences of our failure seriously to study these questions may well be viewed by future generations as our society's greatest injustice to the Negro American.' This is indeed too important a question to be passed over in silence, in the hope that it will solve itself automatically. Will American democracy survive when, as some people fear, the Negro population may have increased from the present 11% to 20% or 25%? However much we may hope that the ethical standard of the American whites will rise correspondingly, we cannot be sure about it. At the time when the slaves were liberated, ethical standards and economic considerations pulled together. They are not pulling together any longer.

Intelligence is not everything, and though the demand for it is still increasing vigorously, it is by no means certain that it will continue for more than perhaps one generation, except in the top brackets. During the technological revolution intelligence became indispensable for production. My feeling is that it may be of equal importance in the future, but for a quite different reason: *in order to understand our civilization, and to be at peace with it.*

THE ETHICAL QUOTIENT

Not many employers would engage a man on the strength of his intelligence alone, without having at least some idea of his honesty. A measure of the ethical character, an 'ethical quotient' or EQ is certainly next in importance after the IQ. There must of course be a great difference between any ethical scale and the intelligence scale. Ethical behaviour is not problem-solving; it cannot be tested by any battery of questions. The Greeks knew that it is no use asking a liar whether he is a liar. Nevertheless, questions are not useless if they are aimed at the views of the individual regarding *others*, not himself. Liars and cheats usually consider all people to be cheats and liars. If somebody thinks that he lives in the jungle, he is likely to be a jungle animal himself, though not necessarily a beast of prey. Reasonably reliable indications can be obtained only from observation of actual social behaviour and this creates another important difference between the IQ and the EQ. The first is a measure that can be applied to school children, the other, properly, only to adults, though the forecasts of experienced educators are often surprisingly accurate. I would regard crime prediction, from tests, heredity and family circumstances at an early age as one of the most important future tasks of psychological science, but this science is still in its infancy. For the present it is an art, instinctively practised by good educators. I believe that they would not have much difficulty in *ranking* their pupils in some such ethical scale as this:

EQ RATING	CHARACTERISTICS OF SOCIAL BEHAVIOUR
130 plus	Dedicated to good works and to the service of others to the point of self-effacement or even self-sacrifice.
120–130	Dedicated to socially useful works, absolute refusal to act anti-socially, but ego not suppressed.
110–120	Socially unimpeachable behaviour, balanced attitude between ego and social environment. Capable of unselfish behaviour.
100–110	Responsible and reliable in the right environment,

EQ RATING	CHARACTERISTICS OF SOCIAL BEHAVIOUR
	but prone to accepting the standards of the majority of his group.
90–100	Good citizen in routine conditions, but capable of mean, selfish acts. Occasional liar.
80–90	Social being under supervision, but capable of occasional dishonesty (not returning excess change, shop-lifting, etc.), poor sense of ethical values, attracted to lower standards, fond of 'kicks'.
70–80	Inclination to envy, hatred, occasional cruelty and criminal behaviour. Prone to fall foul of the law.
70 minus	Brutish, malicious and cruel, habitual criminal.

This is only an *ordinal* scale, suitable for a rough classification of the persons. The final EQ ratings are obtained by *ranking* them in the group, in exactly the same way as in the case of the IQ, that is to say, dividing them into percentiles and distributing them in a Gaussian histogram, with the same standard deviation. If experience with normal groups of young people of sixteen to twenty years shows that my tentative groupings are too narrow or too wide, they should be changed accordingly, to give better guidance.

Note that this is intended to be a *practical* scale. It does not matter whether exemplary social behaviour is motivated by the active love of fellow-brethren, by unconscious inhibition, by vanity, by fear of the police, by the fear of God, or by the love of God. An 'assessment of merit' which takes the motivation into account would be a matter for theologians rather than for social engineers. In the case of people of sixteen to twenty, whose character is already formed, the previous history, heredity, early education, neighbourhood, schooling, etc., is of interest only insofar as it gives some indication of the *stability* of the character to be expected. If the EQ measure were gradually extended to younger age groups, this would be of the greatest interest for recommending corrective education. Heredity, family, etc., are of course also of the greatest interest for the social researcher who wants to disentangle the determining factors of the EQ. The method would be the same as in the case of the IQ: consider subsets with one or other factor fixed or variance-restricted, plot the histogram of the subset, and draw conclusions for desirable reforms.

THE IQ–EQ DIAGRAM

The most important datum with which one can connect the EQ is the IQ, because the IQ measures, roughly speaking, intellectual capability, and it would be of the greatest interest to find out how these two character-components are correlated. The technical procedure is simple. We have now two numbers, the EQ and the IQ of every individual. Let us distribute these as dots in a plane, with the IQ as x-coordinate, and the EQ as y. This gives a two-dimensional histogram, in which we can determine local densities, and draw lines of equal density, enclosing between them certain fractions of the population, for instance 10% as shown in Figure 2. The crux is only that in order to carry this out with acceptable accuracy, one requires very large groups, otherwise the sampling errors in small areas become too large. In the case of the one-dimensional representation there is no great difficulty in fitting the population into a histogram; groups of the order of 100 are sufficient to allot the individuals their right place, except at the tail ends. (In a group of 100, there will be only one individual with 135 plus or with 65 or less, and one does not know exactly where to put these.) In order to construct an IQ–EQ histogram with similar accuracy one requires populations of the order of 10,000, otherwise the histogram will be rather rough.

I have drawn Figure 2 on an assumption which, though fairly likely, need not be true. I have assumed that the joint IQ–EQ distribution is a two-dimensional Gaussian one. This need not be true, because though we have forced the IQs and the EQs *singly* into Gaussian frames, this does not mean that the EQs for *any* given IQ group will have a Gaussian distribution. Deviations from this law, if they exist, would be very interesting. One might find for instance that the feeble-minded (IQs 75 to 50) have a smaller ethical spread than the average. This may make it worth while to undertake the construction of IQ–EQ histograms from very large groups.

The most important conclusion, however, can also be obtained with fair accuracy from smaller groups. This is the question of

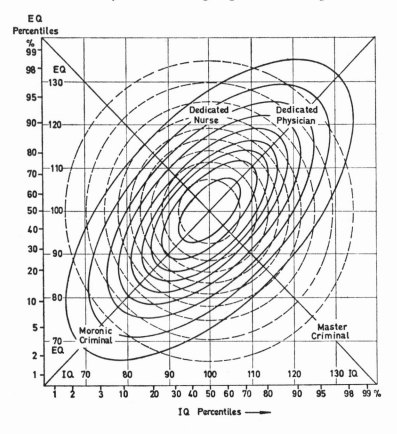

----No correlation, ρ = 0, ——Correlation with ρ = 0·6

Each zone contains 10% of the population

FIGURE 2   *The EQ–IQ diagram.*

the *correlation* between the IQ and the EQ. Mathematically this is defined by a correlation coefficient ρ whose value is between zero and unity. (For the mathematics, see Note 7.) $\rho = 0$ means no correlation between intelligence and ethos; the zones which contain equal fractions of the population become circular.

$\rho = 1$ is the (certainly unrealistic) case in which the IQ completely determines the EQ and vice versa; in this case the whole diagram reduces to a straight line at 45° to the coordinate axes. I have illustrated the not unlikely case $\rho = 0.6$, in which the lines of equal density are ellipses, with an axis ratio of 2:1.

All this might appear as dry mathematics, until we put a few human types into the diagram, such as the 'dedicated nurse', with average intelligence but very high EQ, the 'dedicated physician' with high IQ and EQ,* and two low EQ-types, the 'master criminal' and the 'moronic criminal'. We then realize that *a civilized society would hardly be possible without a rather strong correlation between intelligence and ethos.* If there were no correlation, there would be about as many master criminals as moronic ones. As it is, the master criminal, the great favourite of detective novels (Professor Moriarty, etc.) hardly exists in real life. (Though the four who master-minded the Great Train Robbery in 1963 were far above average intelligence.) Whether one could put Hitler and Stalin into this class is a moot point. Psychometric classifications, which account well for the great majority of people, cannot be expected to provide places for such exceptional phenomena. This is evident also in the IQ scale. On the whole one can expect a good correlation between creativity and intelligence, but the great painter Gustave Courbet and the writers Theodore Dreiser and Knut Hamsun were noticeably lacking in intelligence. Thomas Alva Edison would probably have failed in mathematical examinations.

The question 'Nature or nurture?' raised in relation to the EQ is apt to provoke at least as violent emotions as in the case of the IQ. The liberal conscience is a little too much inclined to put the blame for the crime not on the criminal, but on the society which failed to give him education and chances. Yet we know, since the classical work of the Bavarian jurist Lange in the early years of this century (recently continued by H. L. Eysenck), that there are

* I may have been a little rash in qualifying persons with a high EQ as 'dedicated', because this implies that they are not lazy. I suspect that at the upper end of the scale there is a strong correlation between EQ and dedication. It is difficult to imagine a lazy saint. But it is more exact to say that dedicated doctors and nurses are found *among* certain IQ–EQ pairs.

born criminals just as there are born imbeciles. Statistics on monozygotic (identical) twins have shown that if one of them is in gaol, there is a high probability that the other has also fallen foul of the law at some time; far higher than for the general population, or even for criminals who have dizygotic twins. On the other hand there can of course be no doubt about the influence of a crime-breeding environment, such as is found in slums in general, and in racial slums. Even more than in the case of the IQ it is necessary to approach these problems scientifically and not emotionally. We must obtain *quantitative* knowledge of that part of ethical behaviour which can be influenced by education and by social justice (probably the greater part), and of that part (probably much smaller) which can be influenced only by such questionable means as eugenics, drugs and psychiatric treatment.

COMPLETING THE STATISTICAL DESCRIPTION OF THE DIVERSITY OF MAN

If one asked employers what quality they would appreciate as the third most important after intelligence and honesty, many of them would probably answer without much hesitation: motivation, diligence, industry, stamina. These are not quite synonyms, but they have a strong common component. Society has little use for those who cannot attach their libido, more or less permanently, to some useful pursuit, but soon get bored and disinterested.

But are we justified in considering motivation as a psychological factor of the individual, without specifying *for what* he is motivated? It is really somewhat surprising that this question can be answered, even partially, in the affirmative. There really are people with strong mental energies who ask to be attached to almost anything which is approved by society. But there are also important exceptions. There are for instance highly gifted mathematicians who cannot be interested in anything but pure mathematics. There are also many more people who easily get bored with almost anything, but who, after long search, may discover something which will attract them for a long time. These people are important, because they might represent a danger to the stability of society.

For a moment it might look as if a single factor, whether it is called motivation or diligence, would be useless in itself, unless we split it up into perhaps a thousand branches, according to specific appetites and inclinations. A career adviser cannot of course avoid going into all this in great detail. But it would be premature to conclude that the motivation factor is of no use. Let us assume that the IQ and the EQ of an individual have been already ascertained by respectable psychometric methods. Let him have, for instance, an IQ and an EQ both of 125. These qualify him to become a good medical doctor, a higher administrator, a creative and responsible engineer, etc. If he has no desire to undergo the hard training required for these professions and to lead an exacting life, he is a social misfit. It does not matter that he might find absorbing interest in bridge, in football, in gardening or in women; an employer would have little use for him. I do not think that this would be very different even in a mature society, which need not fully exploit the potentialities of everybody in order to maintain production. Employing people far above or below their IQ and EQ is dangerous.

But how can we ascertain the motivation or diligence of young men or women of sixteen to twenty? Here the near-synonyms part. Diligence can be ascertained only after a long practical trial, but motivation has predictive value. It is possible for an experienced educator or psychological expert to gain a thorough acquaintance with the ideals, values, dreams and wishes of the young man or woman, and to predict from his behaviour during his school years, and also from his family circumstances, whether his attachment to one or the other of his life-plans is sincere and likely to be lasting. This of course is an art rather than a science, and a certain fraction of failures cannot be avoided, but there are people who master this art sufficiently for allotting, say, five marks to different degrees of motivation, such as:

5 Promise of lifelong dedication.
4 Sufficient motivation for success and a satisfied life.

3 Slightly uncertain, but deserves the benefit of doubt, trial of chosen career recommended.

2 Uncertain, deferment of choice recommended.

1 Misfit in his IQ–EQ class, likely to find satisfaction in hobbies rather than in a career.

These motivation numbers now ought to be added to the IQ–EQ diagram, but this would really require a third coordinate, and would destroy its advantage of easy visualization.* As an alternative one could construct five IQ–EQ diagrams, one for each degree of motivation. This would give a more perfect representation of the human material, because a 'dedicated physician', for instance, must not only have a high IQ and EQ, but also strong motivation, hence he would be found in levels 4 or 5. The lower diagrams would represent 'problem children'.

We are now warned that it becomes more and more difficult to increase the number of psychometric factors. (There is no limit to the amount of *individual* psychometric data which can easily be measured in psychological laboratories, but these are hardly of the type of the socially important general factors.) In the case of the EQ we had to rely to some degree on intuition, in the case of motivation even more. Moreover the populations from which significant statistical distributions can be obtained are growing larger and larger. The IQ could reasonably be tested in groups of 100, the IQ–EQ required about 10,000, IQ–EQ motivation about 50,000. Note that if we had 10 psychometric factors, with only 10 levels each, this would give 10^{10} cells, which is about three times more than the whole population of the Earth.

I would like to add, though, a few more general descriptors, which may be of importance for social engineering. The first of these is *dominance*. It has long been known that a 'pecking order' is established in any group of hens, and ethologists, in particular Konrad Lorenz, have found a similar ranking in almost all

* There exists an ingenious method, originated by D. M. MacKay in 1949, for visualizing structures in three or more dimensions by constructing, by means of a computer, their two-dimensional projections on a cathode-ray tube screen and rotating them in all free dimensions, until the viewer gets an intuitive idea of them. See Note 8.

species of animals which live in groups. In a recent book* the distinguished Australian biologist, Sir Macfarlane Burnet, emphasized the fundamental importance of dominance in human society. Indeed, not even the most primitive human societies could have survived without some sort of ranking, which was first one-dimensional and based upon brute force like the pecking order, and later branched out into elaborate hierarchies. Nor will a mature society survive without some sort of vertical order. If the anarchists would succeed in destroying the 'establishment' and creating anarchy, this would soon bring back the dominance of the most undesirable kind – brute force.

A hierarchical structure justified by social usefulness is an indispensable feature of any highly developed society. What we must guard against is 'pure' dominance; the will of individuals to subject others to their power – because they enjoy it. In its extreme form I would call this 'power addiction', and it is my contention that power addicts must be excluded from power in a mature society. 'The meek must inherit the Earth', because the power addicts have been responsible for the greater part of the miseries of mankind. Unfortunately, what we call history is mostly the story of the misdeeds of power addicts. As Aldous Huxley once remarked, what can we expect of a civilization in which more books have been written about Napoleon than on any other figure in history? I would not of course exclude from power the born leaders of men. Thomas Jefferson and Abraham Lincoln had power, and undoubtedly they enjoyed exercising it, but not for the pleasure of subjecting others to their will. The distinction is a subtle one, but not beyond the power of practical psychologists. Experienced educators will have no difficulty in recognizing the incipient power addict, and warning society against him. Recently students have strongly protested against the (more imagined than real) practice of universities passing files on to their prospective employers, which contain records of their political activities. On the other hand it has been universal practice in all armies and most civil services that a description not only of the abilities but also of the character of any member

* Macfarlane Burnet, *Dominant Mammal, The Biology of Human Destiny*, Heinemann, Melbourne, 1970.

of these organizations shall pass from one immediate superior to the next. A system will undoubtedly work best when it has complete information on its members. The individual concerned could of course have access to his file. I can understand the students who would like to play at being subversive without damaging their chances of a good job later in life, and I do not think that political opinions during the youthful years are necessarily a part of the character. But power addiction *is* an aspect of the character, and I believe that society has a right to defend itself against incipient tyrants. In a democratic system they would probably not get very far anyway; a will to power without the other attributes of leadership will soon be resented by colleagues, but even petty tyrants can cause much unhappiness.

The opposite end of the dominance scale, submissiveness or *suggestibility* (the tendency to conform with the values of the personal environment), also has its social dangers. In itself it is neither good nor bad. It is good for those who enter a high-class educational institution, or a religious order, and acquire standards of unselfish behaviour far above the average. It is bad for the gifted boys born into the working class, who imitate their dart-throwing, beer-drinking elders, and dare not distinguish themselves by tastes, language or knowledge. It is extremely bad for those in the slums who join gangs of juvenile delinquents, or for the high-school boys in some Latin-American countries, who join kidnapping and murder gangs led by dominant individuals. Such youngsters will also easily become drug addicts because they will not be able to resist when they are 'dared' to try the drugs, in spite of exhortations from schoolmasters, posters and parents. Suggestibility too ought to be noticed at an early age by the educators, and special care ought to be taken to put such individuals into the right environment.

One more descriptor I want to single out for attention, which will strike many readers as strange: *the capacity for happiness*. In the ancient world it would have been frivolous to talk of this. The Greeks (not, perhaps, all of them) equated happiness with social standing; the highest degree was 'the happiness of kings'. But in the present epoch, when the pressure of scarcity is waning and we are approaching something like social justice, the term is perfectly legitimate, because the happiness of individuals will be more and more limited by their *own* talent for it. We are now living in a sufficiently just and rich society to recognize that people are very differently endowed with this gift. And the most valuable people in a mature society will not be the most productive, perhaps not even the most creative, but those men and women who are themselves happy and can spread goodwill and happiness around them.

I am not talking of orgasm or ecstasy, nor of the proud, grim happiness of the great artistic or scientific creator, but of the simple happiness which makes people smile. We cannot think of a psychometric device which can distinguish the happy smile from a rictus, or from the conventional smile of the English or the orientals, but for a human observer it is not difficult to observe the difference. It is a rare gift. The drug addicts do not smile, the hippies look grim, and I would not attribute the sad fact that among hundreds of young people dancing you can hardly see a smiling face, to a damnable modern convention and to nothing else.

This instinctive happiness is probably to a great part a matter of physical health, in particular of a well-functioning glandular system, and to this extent it is a problem which the medicine of the future will certainly not fail to solve. The psychological factors are not so easily disentangled. Psychologists and psychiatrists are dealing professionally with defective human material; no wonder that even Freud considered mental health as simply the absence of inner conflicts, and was led logically to the 'Death Wish', which tends to resolve all tensions. We must have respect for his deep pessimism, but we must rid ourselves of it.

Psychologists and psychologically-trained social workers have collected ample material on the types of early education which predestine the child to unhappiness, to alcohol, drug-taking or crime. Avoiding these is certainly the alpha of the science of happiness. The omega is still far away. The question of a 'congenital' tendency to happiness has hardly been raised, though every mother who had a 'happy' child and a 'problem child' will believe in it.*

* See Note 9.

A scientific exploration of the sort of ordinary, instinctive happiness, which one could call childish, is certain to come up against resistance, in the first line from those simple souls, still numerous among us, who would ascribe *all* unhappiness to social deprivation and injustice. But these are not the only objectors. When, in his *Brave New World*, Aldous Huxley described a society in which everybody is happy except the rebellious intellectuals, this by no means the worst of all possible worlds was received with angry revulsion by almost all intellectuals. They did not want any of the happiness of babies!

I have respect for the grim, purposeful rebelliousness of intellectuals, for their satisfaction with permanent dissatisfaction. Creative rebels were in the past powerful agents for progress. But are they all creative? Dostoevsky has masterfully described in his *Notes from Underground*★ the sweetness which a non-creative intellectual sucks from the very depths of his misery. This is a pathological type we can do without.

There is not much that I want to propose in a quantitative way regarding the measurement of instinctive happiness. For experienced educators it would not be difficult to rank them, or to allot marks to them, and one may hope for some agreement about such a scale. But the real work starts after the general statistics are established, by factorial analysis. The purpose is clear. We may not be able to create a Great Society, but we can create a happy, smiling society.

★ Other translations have the title *Letters from the Underworld*. Lewis Mumford calls their anti-hero 'a pre-incarnation of Hitler'.

10. EMPLOYMENT IN THE MATURE SOCIETY

No Utopian writer has yet dared to visualize a Cockaigne, a society in which nobody works. The practical, but psychologically rather naïve, Edward Bellamy let people work up to the age of 45 in the industrial army, but at that age, with the exception of a small number of specialists, he released them from all obligations, to live a life of dignified, educated leisure. Aldous Huxley, in 1931, with mass production and the consumer society already under his eyes, wanted to keep everybody at work for $7\frac{1}{2}$ hours a day, until their sudden and painless collapse around 60, with the roses of youth still on their cheeks. Since that time, already long behind us, nobody in the Western countries has attempted a complete Utopia. The glimpses of the future are either horrible, repulsive Dystopias, or, at best, piecemeal attempts at improving this or that unsatisfactory feature of our present world. We have become too much aware of the weaknesses of human nature, which is made more for 'travelling hopefully than for arriving', which will not fit happily into any static system, however benevolently designed. I am not unaware of these difficulties. We are faced with the enormous double task of arresting the growth of the consumer society before it collapses through wars or through existential nausea, and we must change 'human nature', as it now manifests itself, so as to fit into a system in which progress is not measured by the annual growth of GNP per capita.

I can not (and I do not even wish to) visualize anything like a 'final' state, or more realistically, an almost stationary state which lasts long enough for education and bio-engineering slowly to transform the majority of human beings into the highest types of *homo sapiens*, and the highest types into 'supermen'. But I think that I can visualize a *state of transition* towards it. This would still be a 'consumer society' in the sense that it supplies its citizens lavishly with material goods. In addition it also provides them with ample opportunities for education and entertainment. But it also provides them with *work*; enough work to bear their leisure without boredom. It goes without saying that in the next stage of technology no work need be back-breaking or stultifying. Nor need it be Parkinsonian sham-work.

I will assume, for the transitional period, a level of technology not higher than the present, but much better organized. Until such time as the new education (with as little biological intervention as possible) has transformed 'human nature' sufficiently, so that we can trust it not to fall back into the murderous follies of the past or into a dull and sterile decadence, I believe that we must keep up a level of occupation not very different from the present. But though the time occupied need not change much, the distribution of occupations will have to be made, gradually, very different. Instead of driving the consumer society *ad absurdum*, that part of time which is no longer needed for the production of goods will have to be used for the improvement of the quality of life by an immense extension of services, among which education must have a prominent part.

How much time can we spare from production and Parkinsonian administration, and devote to the improvement of the quality of life? This is usually discussed in terms of the hours per working week, on the tacit assumption that the weeks per year and the working years in a man's life remain unchanged. This is not a very good measure, because the time saved may be better used for long holidays, for sabbatical years, for raising the age of entry, or reducing the age of retirement, rather than for long, dull evenings or weekends. It is better to take as a measure the hours per year, and even better, following J. Fourastié,* the

---

* J. Fourastié, *Les 40,000 heures*, Gonthier-Laffont, Paris, 1965. With 4 weeks of paid vacations and two weeks of legal holidays, 46 working weeks p.a., 40 working years per life, of which 3 are sabbatical years, Fourastié's '40,000 hours' give just 24 hours per week; the same figure which I take as the basis of my estimate of 40% saved from sham-productive work at 40 hours per week.

working hours in a man's life. But as the length of the working week is a familiar measure, I will assume that the gain by good organization is equivalent to a reduction of the working week from 40 to 24 hours. Let us note the paradox that such short hours apply only to those in 'gainful occupation'. The working week of a young mother, whom statistics class as 'economically inactive', has been estimated as between 80 and 90 hours.

Is it realistic to believe that the working week in gainful occupations *could* be reduced to 24 hours or less, at a considerably increased rate of production? This is a highly controversial question. The 'congenital optimist' Morris Ernst* concluded by a straight extrapolation, carried out in 1955, that by 1976 the weekly hours of work in the USA will be reduced to 30. On the other hand Landsberg, Fischman and Fisher,† in an impressive statistical survey of future possibilities running to 1000 pages, devote just five lines to this question, and come to a very different conclusion: 'Recent experience carefully interpreted does not suggest any radical reductions in hours worked per week and weeks worked per year for the labor force as a whole. Outside of agriculture, the projection envisages a drop from the current actual work-week of forty hours to just below thirty-seven hours in 2000.' But I am not concerned with what will be, only with what *could be* if production work were reorganized with a view to man-hour efficiency without fear of unemployment. Here again we meet extremely contradictory opinions, especially on the problem of unemployment by automation. Ben B. Seligman‡ heaps data upon data to prove that automation threatens massive unemployment. Charles E. Silberman§ in a book written in the same year, also supported by much statistical material, derides all such fears. Evidently, the fear of unemployment makes automation such an emotionally charged subject, that it is difficult to

---

* Morris Ernst, *Utopia 1976*, Rinehart & Co., New York, 1955.

† Landsberg, H. H., Fischman, L. L. and Fisher, J. L., *Resources in America's Future*, Johns Hopkins Press, 1963, p. 19.

‡ Ben B. Seligman, *Most Notorious Victory – Man in an Age of Automation*, The Free Press, New York, 1966.

§ Charles E. Silberman, *The Myths of Automation*, Harper & Row, New York, 1966.

find an unbiased witness. My late friend, the engineer Anthony Vickers,* was free from this fear because he believed (from his own experience) that redundant workmen could be rapidly retrained, and he also believed that there was no visible ceiling to consumption. So he was not afraid of quoting well-supported figures such as these: A coal-fired power plant of 2400 MW power requires 550 people for operation, 10,000 men for supplying it with fuel. An atomic power plant of the same power requires 600 men for operation, 1100 men for the fuel supply, a saving of 84%. Containerization saves 90% of the dockers, about 70% of the crew of freighters. Note that this is not 'automation' but simple mechanization, with existing techniques. Such figures are exceptional, but if one looks at nothing more than the difference of productivity per man-hour between the most efficient factories and the average in almost any line of product, one must come to the conclusion that a reduction from 40 hours per week to 24 is a very pedestrian achievement, which is within our reach, without any new inventions.†

One may object though, that this concerns only the 'on-line' production workers (it would be inexact to call 'manual' those whose work consists in pushing buttons, like a typist), who are now only a fraction of the labour force, less than half in the UK and in Germany, about one-third in the USA. Can the hours of the office workers be correspondingly reduced? This has been discussed before (in Chapter 4), with the conclusion that when the computer, the most wonderful of labour-saving devices, *really* starts saving labour, we can expect a reduction in office work at least equal to that on the shop floor. We also had an intimation of the tremendous resistance which any such transformation will encounter.

Let us face the problem squarely. We cannot stop automation and mechanization of manual and clerical work, because it is a powerful means for increasing the wealth and well-being of our

---

* Anthony Vickers, *The Engineer in Society*, Proc. Inst. of Mechanical Engineers, **183**, 1968–9, pp. 87–126.

† This would be even more if we included the saving by making 'consumer durables' more durable, and by slowing down changes in fashion, which I have estimated as one-quarter of the industrial effort.

industrial civilization. But if we do not stop automation and mechanization, we cannot stop the lowest intelligence brackets from becoming unemployable on the production line. We then have the choice of bracketing them with the lunatics and feeble-minded, whom our society already maintains at the taxpayer's expenses. If we pay them just enough to live on, as we pay the unemployed, we destroy their purchasing power, apart from making them miserable and forcing a good proportion of them into alcoholism, drug-taking and crime. If we pay them well while they are not taking part in the production process, we create a dangerous attraction for those who have the intelligence to work, but do not like it much, who may well be a large majority. Besides, I do not think that good pay in idleness would be healthy just for the less intelligent, who are least able to make good use of their leisure.

I see only one way out of these difficulties, and this is that we must maintain *full employment* in the transitional period, extending it even to the least intelligent, giving them work in which they can feel useful and keep their self-respect. Extra work must be provided, not by Parkinson's law, but by a great extension of services. Working hours must be reduced only at such a rate that men and women will be able to make good use of their leisure.

Before going further it will be as well to explain what I mean by leisure. Sebastian de Grazia* has proved very convincingly that most Americans have 'free time', in the sense that they are not spending it at their place of work, but hardly any leisure, because they seldom have the feeling that they are following their free will. Without much malice, one can say that they have seen to it that they shall not have leisure. First of all, the commuters, who spend two to three hours per day on the road, watching the car in front and the traffic lights. Yet these people look not at all unhappy. They know at least what to do for two to three hours. If you asked them why they do not live nearer to their working place, they would say that they cannot afford it, that they cannot bring up their children in a town which is

---

* Sebastian de Grazia, *Of Time, Work and Leisure*, New York, 1964. See also the witty and perceptive study by Staffan Burenstam Linder, *The Harried Leisure Class*, Columbia Univ. Press, New York and London, 1970.

changing into a slum (though it is of course changing into a slum because of the flight of the 'better' people). They are right within their own terms. But for a mature society to sweep the problem of free time under the carpet by keeping a great part of the population on the roads for three hours a day (soon perhaps even more) is no better than keeping them busy with Parkinsonian sham-work. Any reasonable solution of the urbanization problem may add another ten hours per week or so to the time saved at the place of work, and will make it more difficult to shelve the problem of leisure which is *activity outside the realm of necessity, freely chosen and rewarding*. For those with a lucky disposition such activity can be of course what might appear to others as hard work.

INTELLIGENCE–OCCUPATION MATRIX

I have tried to make a first shot at a quantitative treatment of the employment problem in the transition period, with the aid of an 'Intelligence-Occupation Matrix' such as shown in the table opposite.* This is a two-entry table or matrix, in which the columns represent brackets of ability or intelligence and the rows represent occupations. The IQ means here 'as tested in the whole population', and one could add 'at an age at which intelligence tests are still meaningful'. It is certainly not an ideal representation of the ability of adults, but we have nothing better. Once EQ and motivation data become available one could improve the fitting of jobs to people, but this would make the discussion rather too complicated.

The rows in the matrix represent occupations, arranged roughly in the order of the intelligence which they require, from scientists, artists and members of the learned professions down to service operatives. The division which I have adopted is not exactly what is found in statistical year-books, but this matters little, so long as we can do no better than guess at the distribution of the IQ in each profession. The bracketed figures are likely

* First published in 'Technology, Life and Leisure', *Nature*, **200**, pp. 513–18, 9 November 1963.

IQ bracket	133·1 +	126·5–133·1	120·7–126·5	113·6–120·7	104·1–113·6	91·5–104·1	73·5–91·5	Sums
% of population	2	3	5	10	20	30	25	
Science, arts, learned professions	1·6	2·0	2·4					6·0
	(1·0)	(1·2)	(1·8)					(4·0)
Higher administration	0·4	0·8	1·0	1·8				4·0
	(0·3)	(0·6)	(1·0)	(3·1)				(5·0)
Education (below 'specialist' univ. level)	—	0·2	1·6	7·0	7·0			15·8
	(0·4)	(0·7)	(1·2)	(2·0)	(0·5)			(4·8)
Clerical	—	—	—	1·0	3·0	6·0		10·0
	(0·2)	(0·2)	(0·6)	(3·0)	(10·0)	(6·0)		(20·0)
Technicians	—	—	—	0·2	2·0	3·8		6·0
	(0·1)	(0·2)	(0·2)	(0·4)	(2·1)	(1·0)		(4·0)
Production operatives (including farming)	—	—	—	—	7·0	11·0	2·0	20·0
	—	(0·1)	(0·1)	(1·2)	(6·4)	(17·0)	(15·0)	(39·8)
Service operatives	—	—	—	—	1·0	9·2	23·0	33·2
	—	—	(0·1)	(0·3)	(1·0)	(6·0)	(10·0)	(17·4)
								95%

The figures in this table are percentages. The upper figures give the fraction in an IQ bracket, in a type of employment in a society such as could be realized by AD 2000. The figures in brackets are likely guesses in a highly industrialized country at the present time, midway between the USA and the UK.

guesses for an advanced industrial country, somewhere between the USA and Britain, with a fairly high degree of social justice. For instance I have assumed that, even at present, there are no high talents with an IQ of over 133 on the shop floor or on farms, no 'mute inglorious Miltons' and very few higher than average talents who are suffering from cultural deprivation. Even these few I wish to shift to higher stations, as shown by the un-bracketed numbers. These numbers are *normative* but they are not arbitrary. They are restricted by the postulate of social justice, and by the requirements of an advanced society.

Social justice requires that nobody should be employed below his intellectual capacity (unless he is an ethical or motivational freak). We must therefore raise every IQ group as high as possible, but not above the ability bar, which is shown by a slanting line. Justice to society requires that nobody shall be raised to a higher status than is justified by his ability. Society can offer only a limited number of places in the higher occupations. It turns out, however, that this can be reconciled quite well with social justice. Nobody above an IQ of 120 need be in any but the three highest occupational levels. There is no difficulty in clearing the 2% or so of people capable of high-standard university education out of the lower levels, from 'clerical' downwards. C. P. Snow has rightly remarked that this will not be an unmixed blessing. We shall find no highly intelligent people at bank counters, post-office counters, or on the shop floor. This is a sacrifice which we must make for social justice. (I hope, though, that there will be enough intelligent policemen. As their total number is now less than 0·5% in all advanced countries, I did not give them an extra row.)*

I have given an extra entry to technicians, although they are only a fairly small fraction of the labour force, because so much nonsense is talked about them. They include draughtsmen and servicemen for computers, television, cars, etc. There are people who believe that the increasingly complicated machines, such as computers, will require an army of highly trained specialists to tend and mend them. But in any reasonable society it will not be necessary to re-design machines every few years because of 'built-in obsolescence', and computers are already eliminating many hundreds of draughtsmen in the 'lofting rooms' of the shipbuilding and aircraft industries. One can expect many more machines which cut out the draughtsmen by supplying data

* Rather optimistically, I have left out the armed forces, who require *all* levels of intelligence, and would not easily fit into such a classification; I have also left out that very important profession in a mature society: entertainers.

directly to machine tools with numerical control. As regards
repair men, this group must indeed have high intelligence so long
as they have to repair scores of different types of radio or television
sets, without instructions, and with nothing but a screwdriver, a
soldering iron and a test lamp. But most modern complicated
computers and electronic instruments carry with them a detailed
book of instructions, and a test set. It has turned out, to the
dismay of benevolent people who hoped that a revival of
craftsmanship would follow from the complication of modern
technology, that the moronic fringe is more capable of mechan-
ically following the instructions and making a good job of it
than the more intelligent, who soon get bored. If we are to
revive craftsmanship, we must go about it in a more direct way.
I have therefore lowered the average intelligence of technicians
in the normative forecast instead of raising it, with a moderate
increase in their numbers.

There is no difficulty with the highly gifted people and the
highest occupations, but all the more in the middle and lower
ranks. I have halved the number of production operatives,
assuming the by no means Utopian figure of 20%, and have cut
the number of clerical workers down to 10% of the labour force,
assuming that Parkinson's Law must have a stop. As I have
assumed full employment of all those capable of employment
down to the feeble-minded level of an IQ of 73·5 (95% of the
whole population), this leaves us with the job of finding satisfactory occupations for about 30% of the labour force, of whom
about one-third are above average intelligence, two-thirds
below it.

Education or the 'knowledge industry' is already the largest
single industry in advanced countries, and it will grow even
larger. I have shifted the above-average surplus intelligences into
'education below specialist university level' which includes also
the people's universities, and all adult, lifelong education. The
rather bold figure of 15·8% of the labour force includes teachers
and students in their sabbatical years. Assuming that about 60%
of the people have three sabbatical years in their working life of
thirty to forty years, this means about 5% students and 10·8%
teachers. I visualize this great army of teachers not as lifelong

professionals, but composed of perhaps one-half volunteers, who after the age of 40, having done fifteen to twenty years in production or service jobs, will be glad to change their occupation, and to devote themselves to younger people. If such a volunteer army could be found (which of course is somewhat hypothetical) it would be possible to establish a 1:1 relationship between adult students and teachers. This would bring us close to the ideal of Rousseau's *Émile*: one tutor for every pupil, with the difference of course that this would be tutoring in the later years, not in the formative ones.

The most important change in the IQ employment matrix is the halving of the production operatives, and the doubling of service operatives, to a full third of the whole labour force. The reduction in the number of the on-line production workers is a natural consequence of progressive technology, and could be stopped only if we either consciously encouraged restrictive practices on the shop floor, or favoured 'ergonomic' improvements at the cost of efficiency. The first is repulsive; we already have too much of it. New machines are often introduced against the resistance of trade unions only on condition that the redundant workers shall stand idly around it. This saves them from unemployment, but not from boredom. Leisure on the shop floor is not a reasonable ideal. On the other hand 'ergonomics', the art of making work agreeable and interesting, deserves the greatest attention. A very remarkable form of this was practised by a great computer factory in France for some years. Each workman assembled a complete unit of a computer, with hundreds of different manual operations, tested it, and signed it in the end, like an artist. The response of the workmen was enthusiastic; they became interested not only in their work but in intellectual matters, and they became excellent pupils of evening classes. Unfortunately this brilliant experiment was stopped after a few years, when the new, almost fully automated factory was completed. I hope that it may find many followers in the coming years, on the way to a mature society. I believe that the figure of 20% operatives will give a wide margin for ergonomic improvements once restrictive practices have been eliminated.

Up to now the greater part of the labour force which has

become redundant on the shop floor has gone into the offices and only a minor proportion into service occupations. What I mean by service is close to the popular concept, but different from that of many labour statistics. The *International Labour Review* for instance divides out only Agriculture and Industry, all the rest as 'services'. I have separated out not only production workers and administrators, but also clerical workers who are not in personal contact with their public. Education is of course a service, but the rest is no less important. One could imagine a highly developed technological society doing its shopping by remote control and taking its holidays in fully automated hotels and cafeterias, but I would not like to live in it. A high-level civilization requires personal service in shops, catering establishments, even in the home, not by machines and not by slaves, but by free people who do it well, and do it with a smile – and not only because they are well paid for it. At present there is still a stigma on personal service. Most girls would prefer to serve a greasy machine rather than a smiling mistress. (Of course housewives and customers in shops, hotels and restaurants will also have to learn to smile. Those who cannot will not be served.) I do not think that it will be too difficult to make people realize that in a world in which the production of material goods has become almost automatic, personal services, like all good human contacts, will have to be revalued. A good shop assistant or waitress ought to have the same social standing as a good nurse.

I do not propose that the large army of service operatives should consist entirely of lifelong professionals. Everybody, except those in the learned professions, such as doctors (who are also service workers), ought to be trained for a service occupation as a side job, to be practised at intervals. American students do this already, and they do not feel degraded. On the other hand, according to many reports, Russian waiters feel degraded, because they serve their customers with studied slowness, and perfect indifference. Here, as in many other things, something seems to have gone wrong in the great socialist democracy.

A distribution of employment such as has been sketched out will be in harmony with a highly developed production industry of a very advanced technology, without the waste on the shop floor and in the offices by restrictive practices, by cutting down administrative and clerical work to a functional minimum. But, even more important – the manpower released will not be used for taking the consumer society *ad absurdum*; it will be used for services, for *improving the quality of life*.

But how can we make the approach to such a new distribution without *dirigisme*, without ordering the various IQ brackets into their appropriate lines of employment? We must ask first, how did the present distribution come about? Certainly not by planning, but by constant conflict between individual and group interests, with a certain adjustment to a level of technology which was always *behind the times*. The factories had to keep some of the redundant labour under the pressure of the labour unions, and because everybody feared, rightly, technological unemployment. Only Sweden had made reasonably adequate provisions for retraining.* The unhealthy growth in the offices was due not so much to any pressure from labour (though the streamlining of offices always meets with strong opposition), as to bad management, in particular the tendency to 'empire-building'. This was perhaps unavoidable in the growth phase, and it will not be easy to stop it, however ridiculous the growth of overhead costs may become in the era of the computer.

There are, it has been said, two non-violent ways for effecting reforms: Thomas Jefferson's principle 'It is a good thing, let us realize it', and Alexander Hamilton's principle 'Make it pay!' A transformation as thorough as that expressed in the figures of the IQ employment matrix can come about only from the combination of the two principles. The governments and the leaders of opinion must be convinced that it is a good thing, they must prepare re-education and retraining plans, and must enlist the support of those concerned. But they must also make it pay for the individuals and for the interest-groups. The reduced number of workmen and office staff will make production more

* In 1970, 100,000 Swedish workers who had become redundant or were in danger of becoming redundant have been retrained, in six-month courses, paid by the State, and 80% of these immediately obtained jobs in their new profession. In addition more than 50,000 have undergone voluntary retraining in evening classes. I am indebted to Minister Moberg for this information.

efficient, while the market will remain stable, because the redundant workers will not be unemployed, and will retain their purchasing power. Instead of paying for people to be idle on the shop floor and for inflated offices, the taxpayer will pay for larger educational institutions, and he will receive services which were formerly reserved for the minority. Of course this will take time. One cannot make a good waiter out of a redundant miner (though there are some experienced people who dispute this), and one cannot quickly make a good teacher of an old bureaucrat, even if as a young man he had the intellectual and ethical qualifications. Like most reforms, this will work out properly only in the second generation. But come it must, because the alternatives are both ridiculous and frightening.

II. ECONOMIC PATHWAYS TO THE MATURE SOCIETY

For some years after the Second World War the industrial countries in the non-communist part of the world prospered as never before. Did the 'invisible hand' which gently leads private interests towards public goals, and which failed so conspicuously in the decade before the war, start functioning again? Let us not forget that the depression which followed the First World War, was avoided after the second by such 'unsordid' and 'uncapitalistic' acts as Lease-Lend and Marshall Aid. But we must also concede a good part of the credit to free enterprise, which admittedly operated under extremely auspicious circumstances. Germany and Japan were destroyed, but the war had also destroyed their paranoiac political systems and released their technological and economic potential. Italy, which also had to suffer great destruction, no longer aspired to the status of a great power, and like its former allies, did not have to maintain a crippling military establishment. For many years there was a seller's market; it was the epoch of the *Wirtschaftswunder*, the economic miracle. The United States, which until the war was a capital-importing country, had become at last strong in capital, and realized that she could support not only her own rapidly growing industries, but also those of Europe and Japan.* All

---

* Have the States gone too far? In August 1971, at the time of the 'dollar crisis' economists were very divided in their opinions as regards the remedy, but they seem to have been agreed on the point that it was wrong of the USA to have overspent on current account to the extent of some 50 billion 'paper dollars', and to incur such an enormous debt. But the American manufacturers would have been only too happy to supply goods for these paper dollars! Or,

this went *pari passu* with a powerfully improving technology, which paid richly for an unexampled stream of money directed into research and development. Everything seemed to be headed towards an epoch of undreamt-of prosperity and contentment, without any fundamental change in the system and its values.

Now, 25 years later, the picture is much less satisfactory. In Britain and in the United States we have reached the new stage of 'stagflation' – stagnation with inflation. This is a timely warning of more serious troubles to come, which stem from the inability of the free-enterprise system to adapt itself quickly enough to the requirements of a prosperity near saturation, with its attendant psychological distresses. Private and public interests no longer pull smoothly together. In the United States large railway companies are bankrupt at a time when they ought to be able to spend heavily on high-speed electric trains. On the other hand it still pays the motor industry to put more and more cars on the road, to choke the traffic and spread the suburbs wider and wider, while the centres of many big towns change into slums. Almost every large town has plans for underground railways which have been shelved because there is no money for them, while the roads are jammed with cars and clouded with exhaust fumes. It still pays to put office skyscrapers into big towns, to make the traffic worse; it does not pay under the rent control system to rebuild the inner, decaying parts of cities, let alone to construct planned, self-contained new towns. Savings flow into modern South Sea Bubbles; there is never enough money for slum clearance. And it still pays (though, let us hope, not for much longer) for chemical manufacturers to pollute the air and the seas.

Where private vested interests are obviously opposed to public welfare, it is evident that the power of the central authorities

---

if their rules had allowed them, the central banks could have bought a share in the American industry. (The 40 billion dollars which they held between them are less than 1% of the US industrial capital.) What, with our monetary conventions, appears as a 'dollar crisis' is, more realistically, a crisis in the international distribution of employment. For many years the USA has supported employment abroad, at the cost of its own. We talk of a scarcity of gold, while we suffer really from insufficient employment to go round.

must be strengthened – but is this not the way to the all-powerful, totalitarian state? To a stiff, sluggish, central bureaucracy, to progress slowed down by the lack of self-interest? I hate all such extrapolations. Such warnings most often come from people for whom free enterprise means carrying on their business tomorrow as it was yesterday. Our democratic civilization is built on compromises, and I do not see why we should not adopt a reasonable compromise which reconciles the liberal belief in the energy of the individual with goal-settings in the public interest.

I have quoted above a few examples in which it does not pay for private capital and for independent industrial firms to steer towards the public welfare. The democratic solution to such problems is: 'Make it pay!' This does not mean that we must make 'lame ducks' solvent, or that we ought to pay for pollution control out of public subsidies. There is no need always to make up the difference with taxes. If plastic bottles or waxed-paper cartons present an insuperable disposal problem, the public will be quite willing to go back to glass bottles. They can be made to pay for electric motor cars in towns, when internal combustion engines are prohibited. Smokeless zones have been established in many big towns, without any great rise in taxes or rates. Tolls can be introduced on the motorways on a level at which the railway companies can make the competing fast electric trains pay their way. Of course it is the public who will have to pay for all this; but the public will get clean air and safety in exchange. Is it not worth paying a little more for transport to save some tens of thousands of road deaths and hundreds of thousands of cripples? The hospital and repair charges for motor car accidents would, by themselves, constitute a handsome subsidy for safe, fast electric railways, without counting the lives saved.*

There are other establishments in the public interest where it is not so easy to raise the capital without using the taxpayers'

---

* In Britain the Road Research Institute estimates the social cost of a person killed as £8300 ($20,000); in the States the corresponding figure would be about $50,000. In the USA 55,000 people are killed every year on the roads. If by fast and safe public transport this number could be reduced by only 10,000 it would represent a saving of $500 million, which is quite comparable with the losses of $400 million suffered in 1970 by the Penn Central Railroads.

money. In most highly industrialized countries the expenditure of the public sector is now about one half of the GNP. (Britain and France are leading with 53% and 46%.) In the European countries a considerable part of this is raised as health and old-age insurance. I have no doubt that nationalized health services were necessary and beneficial, but they were necessary only because of a cultural lag. If in the European countries the peoples had been asked by a plebiscite whether they wanted a national health service or preferred to keep the money in their pocket, it is probable that they would have voted down the health service with a considerable majority. But a good many of this majority would not have voluntarily laid aside a sufficient sum for medical service and dental care, not even those who could have afforded it. Only a prosperous population, educated for responsibility, could be trusted to pay their part of a health service which amounts to 6 to 8% of all personal expenditure, so that these services would be free only for the poor and the aged. This would have been desirable, because *responsibility is a psychological necessity*. It is now too late for this, and heavy taxation, for health services and free social insurance for all, will make it more difficult to finance such vitally important plans as better public transport, new towns, slum clearance and a greatly intensified and extended educational system.

Let us clarify what financing means. Our economic system is based on the recognition of credit, though the principle has been much eroded by permanent inflation; credit is seldom repaid in full. Financing means, in elementary terms, the exchange of one sort of credit for another. In practice it is far from being so simple. Banks can create credit by an act of will, within certain limits, one can say *so long as the credit is credible*. This brings into the question a psychological element which nobody even claims to have fully understood. At the present time, when all countries have gone off the gold standard, this applies *a fortiori* to international credits. There comes a point at which the exchange rate of currencies is no longer credible, and speculators make a run on them.

At the time of writing there is a confusion which could hardly be worse. In the USA and in Britain the governments and the central banks are trying to restart the economic machinery, which has come almost to a stop, but they have had to restrict credit in order to prevent runaway inflation. Only the near-desperate situation which arose in August 1971 could force the US Government to introduce, as a temporary measure, wage and price controls, which have not yet functioned well in any country. At the same time a school of economists are advocating a great extension of credit and deficit budgets, in order to create the demand which, they hope, will bring back economic growth without excessive inflation. Governments will probably be forced to go this way, by public pressure, but it is unlikely that they will be able to slow down inflation without arresting the inflation-preserving mechanism – the leap-frogging wage demands of the unions, who by anticipating inflation maintain it. The employers, who do not want strikes or go-slows, grant the union demands, but as they do not want to go bankrupt they raise their prices, and so the vicious circle goes on and on. It is a moot point who is leading; each side is accusing the other. Evidently the feedback loop could be cut at either point, by wage restraint *or* by price control; but for psychological reasons it can only be broken, if at all, at *both* points simultaneously. The story of runaway inflation in the past is encouraging; there comes a stage at which everybody gets tired of it, and then the governments and the central banks can stop it without violent reaction.

But even if, as is to be hoped, the present stagflation can be ended, soon or in a few years, and the flow of credit starts again, private money will of course flow into those channels which in the past have proved profitable. Some of this will have highly beneficial effects. By improving its equipment, industry may be able to make good its delayed growth in productivity, perhaps even to catch up with the increasing unwillingness of the workers to work a full week, which now manifests itself in voluntary absenteeism. It may be possible to effect a great overall reduction in working hours, without a loss in material comfort. But there is no reason to expect that private capital will flow to any greater extent into better public transport, planned urbanization, hospitals, habitations for the aged and great new plans for education, unless these are made to pay.

Are such grandiose plans at all realistic? Many people will be inclined to ask: 'Where is the money to come from?' To which I would reply with the question: 'Where is the money coming from to pay the millions who are now paid for doing nothing?'* Those for example who stand on the shop floor, around a machine which has made them redundant; the millions in the offices who are circulating unnecessary papers from desk to desk. If we can pay these people while they are actually producing nothing, why could we not pay them when they are building new towns, etc., or while they are retraining for new jobs, such as teaching and other services?

The labour, the materials and the know-how are available for all this; they can be spared from the sham-work without damaging the economy. *Economically*, that is to say in terms of materials and services, the transformation is possible, therefore it must be also possible to finance it. The first step towards this is the admission that our system is not as efficient as many like to believe. The employers will be more willing to admit this than the unions, both the manual and the clerical. But if it were possible to convince them that increased efficiency does not mean unemployment, we may reach the second stage – public consent. The third stage is financing, *without inflation*. Previously I have mentioned a few problems which can be solved by making it *not pay* to follow bad practices, such as pollution or putting more motor cars into congested areas. I am not in favour of too many such punitive practices. I would prefer positive inducements.

Let us (perhaps optimistically) assume that the resistance of the labour unions can be overcome if there are large programmes which offer new jobs to the redundant workers. Industrial (and many commercial) firms will then be only too happy to speed up the streamlining or 'cybernation' process, which is now going on at a slow rate. They will have no difficulty in raising the capital required for modernization in the open market, because they can confidently expect lower overhead costs at increasing outputs.†

* If I remember well, I have heard this picturesque expression first from the British industrialist, Sir Iain Stewart.

† There is a difficulty, though, which I do not want to leave unmentioned. In any sane, maturing society the output will not increase indefinitely. Until now hope was so closely tied up with growth, that with few exceptions only those industries modernized which could expect a rapidly expanding market.

But how to raise the capital for the public programme, new towns, fast electric railways, schools, hospitals, etc., which do not promise profits, but only social benefits? Many contemporary thinkers have thought of approaching this problem by a 'cost-benefit analysis' which converts social benefits into profits for the community. Such a scale may indeed be useful when it is a question of deciding between different programmes, but it does not solve the problem. In a free economy a socially beneficial programme can compete with profitable ones only it if can be made to show a profit for individual enterprise, otherwise the capital has to be taken out of the pockets of the taxpayer. I believe though that there is an intermediate way. Take the profit out of taxes but not the capital. Let the State issue a new type of bond for the financing of public works, not with a fixed value, but redeemable according to the index of industrial shares, and not with a fixed interest, but with a rate tied to the market value. This will be an attractive proposition for those who want to invest their money safely rather than speculatively. The dividends of course will have to be paid by the taxpayer of the future, but who can pay for the future if not the future? The taxpayer of the future will enjoy, in return, the social benefits. Of course, many safeguards will have to be provided that the State shall use the capital wisely for works of social benefit, and not for hordes of more civil servants. So far the safest way of doing this is to farm out the projects to large private firms, who can be trusted to be efficient, and who in turn are under supervision by ministries, or by parliamentary committees.

The way which I suggest can be characterized in terms which I

Bertrand de Jouvenel has expressed this forcefully: 'L'idée d'une économie stationnaire quant à ses fruits et progressive quant à ses méthodes est un monstre intellectuel.' (*Arcadie*, Futuribles, Paris, 1968, p. 30.) Also: 'L'augmentation de la puissance productive . . . est tellement essentielle à notre société que celle-ci risquerait de s'effondrer au cas d'un tel relâchement.' (*Ibid*, p. 60.) This is indeed a serious danger. We can counter it only by breaking the fatal tie between hope and growth and by inculcating the ideal of *excellence* instead of quantitative growth into our industrial elite. If we fail to break this tie, the industries close to saturation might be struck by premature sloth.

borrow from J. Rivoli:* Keep as much as possible of the public programme inside the *market* economy, and keep the *administered* economy to a minimum. Only a minimum is to be raised by taxes and other forced contributions. This, I believe, is the best way for utilizing the energies of a free society.

There are of course difficulties which are not financial. Making hundreds of thousands of workers mobile, who have settled down comfortably near the factories where they are becoming redundant, and putting them on the road to build new towns, is not an easy operation. Spontaneously, they would much rather settle down in or near to a Megalopolis. There exists now, as in the time of Ricardo and Marx, an 'industrial reserve army'; but this does not consist of unemployed navvies who are willing to go anywhere, and sleep under tents, or even on the ground. Many might be willing to move though, if they were given comfortable trailers, or motor homes.† The motor car industry would be happy to provide them, if somebody would pay for it, so this is again a question of financing. But a great number of redundant workers would be unwilling to undergo retraining for a new job, even in their own town; their monotonous job has generated in them a mental inertia which could be overcome only by a coercion that I would not propose to apply.‡ This

---

* J. Rivoli, *Vive l'Impôt!* Le Seuil, 1965, p. 22, quoted by Bernard Cazes, *La Vie Economique*, Armand Colin, 1965, p. 66. The division between the private and the public sector need not at all coincide with that between the market and the administered economy. Only the last must be financed by taxes.

† In the United States there are already 600,000 families with 'mobile homes'.

‡ Retraining the meat packers in Armour & Co., Chicago, and in many other US firms has proved so unsuccessful that Max Horton, Michigan's Director of Employment Security, gave vent to his feelings in 1961 in the words: 'I suppose that it is as good as any way for getting rid of the unemployed – just keeping them in retraining. But how retrainable are the mass of these unskilled or semi-skilled unemployed? Two-thirds of them have less than high school education. Are they interested in retraining? But, more important, is there a job waiting for them when they have been retrained? The new California Smith-Collier Act retraining program drew only 100 applicants in six months.' (Quoted by Donald A. Michael, *Cybernation, The Silent Conquest*, Center for the Study of Democratic Institutions, Santa Barbara, 1962.)

On the other hand the Swedish retraining programme operates very satis-

psychological obstacle can be overcome, if at all, only by an educational system which does not allow middle-aged workers to become 'old dogs, who cannot learn new tricks'. We cannot therefore expect such a considerable redeployment as I have sketched out in Chapter 10 to become fully successful in less than about one generation. At the start it would come up against psychological resistance not only in the case of unskilled and semi-skilled workmen, but perhaps even more in the case of clerical staff, many of whom have become just as dull and mentally lazy at the desk, as the others on the shop floor. But allowing for all this, I expect that there would be from the start a considerable army of 'volunteers', willing to undergo a change of jobs. Moreover, a large number of the workers who are needed for the great new public programmes need not leave their working places. The same great firms which now build redundant office skyscrapers could start building human habitations. These great firms have cornered a considerable part of the talent and energy-pools in the non-communist nations, and these valuable people must be utilized, without turning them into civil servants.

The first steps towards the mature society, which I have tried to sketch out, are far from revolutionary. They presuppose a society which is devoted to work, but which provides for its leisured future as the good citizen of today tries to provide for his old age. It is a society which saves and invests, and is therefore a capitalistic society, but which has eliminated the 'free-for-all' fight that now produces such painful conflicts between private and public interests. The heroic age of capitalism is long past. Bertrand Russell writes that the old history of British railways reads like the story of romantic robber barons, but some fifty years ago, before nationalization, the boards of the railway companies consisted of sleepy peers and widows. They went to sleep a little too early, and it was only nationalization that brought British railways up to a modern standard – still far from what is technically possible and socially desirable. In the United

---

factorily, though the Swedish population has a lesser tradition of mobility than the American. One cannot help attributing this to the much superior Swedish educational system and to the determined guidance of the Government. (See footnote on p. 98.)

States, where nationalization is taboo, the railway companies will have to rejuvenate themselves, but they cannot do this without new legislation, and some such aid in raising capital as I have tried to outline. They will never be independent again, as they were a hundred years ago, but this does not mean that they will be managed by an inefficient bureaucracy. They will always have the State as a partner, but the example of Japan shows clearly enough that this need not suppress individual energies. Ownership and managership have long separated. The American manager can still build up for himself a moderate fortune, but though this may be important for him as a measure of success, it is far from being the source of his drive. For such people the primary drive is towards an *achievement*; building up a great, live smoothly operating establishment. Financial reward is a very secondary consideration. Of course 'empire-building' can be a very dangerous disease of the social body. When properly directed, it can be the source of its greatest strength.

For a generation, or perhaps two, in the age of transition towards a mature society, we must make use of high-energy individuals, and play the economic game more or less according to the traditional rules, but there can be no doubt that during this time interest in the economic drive will gradually fade out. Once the new education has inculcated *responsibility* into everyone, without the straitjacket of the age of scarcity, the economy can be allowed to become as smoothly efficient and imperceptible as the water supply of big towns used to be before the increasing danger of modern pollution. What will the high-energy individuals do then? We need not worry; the management of restless, Irrational Man will never be easy!

12. THE FAMILY AND EARLY EDUCATION

In this and the next three chapters I will try to sketch out my views on the type of education necessary for a stable and progressive mature society. I am fully aware of the difficulty of the task. My knowledge is inadequate, but so too is contemporary knowledge, judging from the welter of contradictory opinions among professional educators. We are faced with a problem which has never been solved; how to prevent a successful society from falling into decadence?

We can leave aside the naïve idealism of the early socialists and anarchists: that Man is intrinsically good, and that his nature has been corrupted by such institutions as private property and state power. We can equally disregard those who believe that Man is a wild animal, that will never be tamed. The fact is that Man's diversity ranges from the saint to an extremely dangerous and cruel beast. How much of this is congenital and how much is determined by education and environment is an open question. I have no doubt that one generation hence we shall be able to answer it much better than today. One of the many socially useful applications of computers will be the sorting out of influences and their effects in millions of individuals. The input to these will require an army of trained psychologists, who will fill in test records of high complexity. I have little sympathy with those who protest against this in the sacred name of privacy. The lives of the great creators, of a Beethoven or Leonardo da Vinci, have been analysed in intimate personal detail; why should this be forbidden in the case of the common man? Anyway, the information will not be made public. Most of it will go straight into computers for factor analysis and storage. If particularly interesting individual records are published they will be, like medical case-histories, anonymous.

It is my contention that the mature society must be an open, free society, otherwise it will not be capable of development, and will not deserve to exist. To this extent it must be also a permissive society, though we must be somewhat cautious with the interpretation of this fashionable term. At present it means mostly the rejection of the sexual standards of the older generation, but, more dangerously, it means also the denial of its chief values and habits: achievement, work, deferred gratification, and the rejection of an education which tries to impose these values on the young. If we yield to this pressure, the result can be nothing but disorder, leading to a collapse, and in the end to a totalitarian society. A permissive society can exist only if coercion is replaced by inner discipline, by a sense of responsibility, and this must be imparted by the right sort of education. The more permissive a society, the less can it do without a hard apprenticeship. This is an old wisdom; all successful societies have applied it, often to excess. There must be an element of hardship in education, but we must learn to keep it down to the unavoidable minimum, otherwise we might achieve the opposite. As an English judge has remarked in a celebrated murder case, an ultra-ethical, sectarian education is the best breeding ground for criminals. The children of brilliant, highly ethical parents often turn out to be the worst failures. Examples are abundant, but too painful to be mentioned by name. As everywhere in this book, I am for compromises.

In brief, I believe in a loving, permissive early education in the family to perhaps the age of six, and in an education to responsibility after that to the age of perhaps eighteen, which must contain an element of hardship. By that age, however, social responsibility must be sufficiently inculcated, and a certain measure of effort must be made to become a habit, so that the university years, at least for the great majority, can become an introduction to the permissive society.

Until fairly recently, most psychologists agreed that the first five to six years were the real formative years, after which the character sets 'as in plaster'. The newer school of psychoanalysts, in particular Erich Fromm and Erik Erikson, dispute this, and there is much to be said for their arguments. But though the first years of life may not be as all-important as Freud and others believed, they are certainly very important. In the past most children spent their early years with their father and mother, though the number of foundlings brought up in orphanages has at times approached 20%. With the improved expectation of life orphans have now become comparatively rare. The proportion of illegitimate births in Britain has risen from 4% at the beginning of the century to about 9% now, but hardly any of these children will be handed over to orphanages, and only a fraction of them will be adopted. There is an increasing tendency for the mother to retain them, which means that they will grow up without a father. This certainly has its dangers, because the children are likely to grow up with a hatred of the father who disowned their mother, and might transfer this hatred to other males.

In the Industrial and Post-industrial Society the family is in danger. It is no longer a solid economic unit, as it was in the pastoral and agricultural civilizations. It is not held together by property which must be transmitted, nor by the economic dependence of women, nor by strict secular or religious laws. The sacredness of an exclusive, lifelong union has been much weakened by 'instant sex'. For my part, as I wrote in my first book, I would wish for the revival of the multi-generation family house, grouped around property and enriched by the perennial nature of a family, which in past times was the privilege of the rich, perhaps their most enviable privilege. I have little hope, though, of this becoming the norm of life. But however little one expects of the family of the future, one ought to expect that it will hold together until the children are grown up. A good nursery may be better than a broken home, but a good home is better than the best nursery.

There is a fair agreement among psychologists that loving parental care in the first years of life is most likely to give men and women emotional security and stability in later life. It is not without its dangers; all love is likely to go to extremes of possessiveness and exclusiveness, and the Oedipus complex may well leave behind slowly-healing scars. I believe that it is worth accepting this danger, because those who have enjoyed love in their early childhood will be able to give love, and to receive it.

It is likely that the prurient searchlight which publicity is casting on the sex life of the young gives us a highly distorted picture of the modern young family. In all probability it is still better than in the rich Victorian families, where the children were entrusted to nannies, or in the poor families, with a tired father who came home only to eat and to sleep, and an overworked mother, ignorant even of the rules of elementary hygiene. In all probability, most children now born in the industrial countries, except perhaps in the diminishing slums, are *wanted* children. (Perhaps 80% in all.) There is, however, a noticeable tendency towards children being born to parents at an age at which they are not yet psychologically ready for them. They may be a minority, but in our world even a small minority of unstable persons can give trouble far beyond their numbers.

My conclusion is, that *education for parenthood* must be a compulsory subject for every adolescent boy or girl, before they leave school. They must be made deeply aware of the responsibility which they will bear for the happiness of their children. Not every man or woman is cut out to be a good parent. A frightening number of them 'take it out' on the children. In a single year in Britain 40,000 cases of cruelty by parents to children have been brought to court, and this is certainly only a fraction of the number committed. As I heard from a lady doctor in a children's ward, very often a child is brought to the ward with terrible injuries – 'little Johnny has fallen down the stairs' – when it is clear that the child has been cruelly beaten, but the hospital staff are reluctant to denounce the parents. If all the unworthy ones, and not just the emotionally unstable, could be dissuaded from becoming parents, it would be easier to cope with the imperative that a stationary society can allow only about 2·3 children per couple. The voluntary elimination of those unfit for parenthood would allow more children for those who are 'parentally gifted'.

Young, educated middle-class women are already devouring by the million books on the 'care of the baby' and on child psychology. This knowledge will have to be brought home to all. And those women fit for it must be encouraged to give all their time to their children in their formative years, instead of unloading them on nurseries. An advanced technological society has no need of the productive work of all young women. There is no need for them to rush back to their machines or typewriters. After the children have grown up, there is no necessity to fill the great emptiness with routine occupations learned before the first child was born. The great emptiness will be better filled by the first course in adult education, by preparing for a new profession, or by absorbing that 'useless' culture which the young girl may have judged 'irrelevant'. The mature woman of thirty to forty-five may be ready for it.

For the young father the most important part of his educative work starts a little later, and ends later, if it ends at all. Most boys have a natural inclination to admire their father, and a cultural gap between father and son is painful for both. The middle-class father who at nights studies the encyclopedia in order to be able to answer his son's questions makes us smile a little, but we ought to admire him. For such fathers this may be an introduction to lifelong education. In an environment which values knowledge for its own sake he will not put down the encyclopedia with a sigh of relief when the son has grown up, but will want more of it.

Early childhood, as Melanie Klein has emphasized, is a period of strong emotions and infantile rages. No parents, however patient and permissive, can always provide instant gratification for the howling baby, and they would be wrong if they did. But on the whole it is a permissive phase in the education, with only an unavoidable minimum of frustration, and almost no effort is expected from the willpower of the child.

A permissive education can mean very different things. One extreme was the education of the infant James Stuart Mill, who sat with his books in the working room of his father James Mill, and was free to interrupt him with questions at any moment. This is not a bad method for outstanding intellects. But for the average child permissive education means that he is allowed to play, and to learn only by his natural curiosity. The success of the infant schools founded by Maria Montessori is now beyond a question. The 'absorbent mind' of the child takes in the grammar of very complicated languages, or even two languages at a time, without any systematic schooling.

At the present time there is a strong educational movement for introducing the methods of Maria Montessori, reinforced by the researches of Jean Piaget, on the processes by which the infant forms its world-picture, to an age group for which these were not originally intended, between six and twelve years. The movement started a little over ten years ago in England, where now more than one-third of the primary schools are reported to have adopted the 'Open Plan', and is now rapidly spreading in the United States. In these schools there are no classrooms in which the children sit on benches and listen to the teacher. There are no desks, but tables with educational toys with which the children teach themselves to weigh, count and read, if they wish they can sculpt, draw and paint, or just tumble and romp about in the corridor. They differ, however, from the now defunct American 'progressive' schools in the burden which they throw on the teacher. The teacher is supposed to go round, compliment-ing each child on what it has achieved and leading it on to the next stage, to more recondite exercises, to writing on a black-board, even to reading books. It is claimed that the children are not only much happier than in the old 'formal' schools (which is not surprising), but they show also better intellectual development. One American school in a ghetto district claims that 99% of the children could read after the first year, something which had never been achieved before.

One cannot help being a little sceptical about these claims. Almost any educational reform works at first, because it is started by the best and most enthusiastic teachers. One can accept the outstanding results claimed for children from culturally deprived homes; the formal schools often failed to establish any contact with them. An expert assures me that ghetto children prefer to be taught by audio-visual machines rather than by a teacher against whose authority they have a strong emotional resistance. But when it comes to children gifted above the average, from homes which are not culturally deprived, one cannot help feeling that an extension of the play period in life to eleven or twelve is artificial and unfair. At this stage it is time to train the willpower of the child, and to let him acquire knowledge which cannot be assimilated without an effort.

13. HARDSHIP AND COMPETITION

Philosophers of all eras have agreed that man cannot be permanently happy. Those who pretended to deny this, the Cynics and Stoics, admitted it too, in a defeatist way. The practical teaching of the Greek Cynics and Stoics, and also of the Tao ('The Way') can be summed up in a few words: 'Do not desire, and you will not be disappointed. Do not try, and you will not fail.' Some Existentialists have said much the same, in millions of confused words.

Why can man not be permanently happy? Is this perhaps foreshadowed in every nerve, in which a steady stimulus, continued for a long time, either becomes unnoticed, or changes into unendurable pain? This would be a far too sweeping conclusion. Animals have the same sort of nerves as we, but some of them can be permanently happy. Anybody who has seen sea-lions or dolphins at play cannot doubt that these are happy creatures and we are not surprised when we read of their almost incessant lovemaking. But how can we know that they are happy? I would say that even a solipsist philosopher knows when his dog is happy, though he may be in doubt about his wife, and even more about himself. 'Ask yourself whether you are happy and you cease to be so,' wrote John Stuart Mill in the period of doubt which attacked him around the age of twenty.* He exaggerated a little. There *are* some permanently happy men and women in this world, though far too few. There are some who jump out of bed in the morning with a gay shout, looking forward to the work and pleasures of the day. There are unfortunately many more who are in permanent pain.

* J. S. Mill, *Autobiography*, 1873.

J. S. Mill wrote also: 'If the reformers of society and government would succeed in their objects, and every person in the community were free and in a state of physical comfort, the pleasures of life, being no longer kept up by struggle and privation, would cease to be pleasures.' Which did not prevent him from remaining a noble utilitarian liberal, and from working on social reforms to the end of his life. We must follow his example.

For us, who have tasted progress, a world free from desires, or satiated, is not worth thinking about. The Greek Stoics lived in an epoch of decadence, in which all change was feared to be for the worse, the Chinese Taoists in a timeless, stagnant society, stable but not enviable.* The Mature Society need not be stagnant, except in population and in GNP. It must preserve the value of success achieved by effort, and it must therefore know unsatisfied desires and frustration. Perhaps some time it may become possible to breed that rare type of man and woman for whom life is a happy play, and who for their total physical and mental equilibrium need no contest more serious than a game. I am very much in favour of encouraging *homo ludens*, and I do not believe that he need be sterile and uncreative. But taking humanity as it is, I do not think that we can do without hardship and competition, at any rate for a long time.

Most savage civilizations have instinctively recognized the social value of hardship; what we would call *wanton* hardship, added to what they had to suffer by necessity. One would think that it is no great honour to be an adult warrior in a tribe of Red Indians in North America, or of a tribe of Indios in the Amazonas region, but for them it is a great and cherished honour, because it is acquired at a high price. To this day the initiation ceremony of the Indios consists in flogging the candidate from head to foot, and then sticking maddened insects on his back. Far be it from me to recommend such barbarity, but we must not be blind to the psychological principle behind it. The barbarous initiation ceremonies assured the survival of the Indians and Indios in an

---

* The Chinese world was timeless at both ends, there was not only no end to it, but no beginning. It is astonishing that while almost all primitive peoples have some myth about the creation of the world, however childish, the highly gifted Chinese had none.

environment in which the food (by no means daily food!) could be obtained only by incredibly tough hunters. The Spartan hardships allegedly recommended by Socrates in Plato's *Republic* were also justified by the need for survival of a nation between envious, hostile neighbours. But I contend that a measure of hardship, intellectual rather than physical, is just as indispensable in a highly developed mature society, not threatened by outer enemies. A society in which all desires are satisfied from the cradle to the grave, without an effort, is bound to become decadent.

The sound puritanical instinct of the English upper classes has created a civilized counterpart of the initiation ceremonies of the savages in the great Public Schools. The similarity was more pronounced in the 19th century (around 1820) when Dr Keate, the Headmaster of Eton, became notorious as a sadistic 'flogger'.* Today corporal punishment has largely been abolished, but in certain schools pupils still sleep in unheated rooms, wash in ice-cold water, and often have cross-country runs before breakfast. To have been a public schoolboy is no longer a sufficient or necessary qualification for a distinguished position in England, the Commonwealth or the Colonies, yet many middle-class families still make painful sacrifices for an expensive education, which they could have for nothing in the State schools, because it makes 'gentlemen' of their sons. And I consider the English gentleman as not a bad model for the citizen of the mature society.

Hardship alone, of course, will not do it. In the Kaiser's Germany the only schools which imposed a similar Spartan regime on their pupils were the cadet schools of the officer class, and these were imitated, with even more emphasis on hardship, by the Nazi schools for the SA and the SS. They achieved their purpose – but what a purpose!

While the English Public Schools were early leaders in impart-ing civic virtues by physical hardship and the enforced closeness of the pupils, the French *lycée* can be seen as the leader in education for competitiveness. These, with the French elite universities (the *Grandes Écoles*) and their system of hard competitive examina-

* See Note 10.

tions, have created an admirable elite for governing a people who are not as easy to govern as the English, because they have so much less of the puritanical strain. The French system has been much weakened by the great extension of university education after the war, and after the student riots of 1968 its efficiency is in some doubt.

Education in a mature society must combine a measure of hardship for all, with competitiveness for the elite. I repeat, people do not appreciate what they receive without effort, and the membership of the consumer society is no exception. The super-abundant industrial civilization of the future will supply almost free many goods and services which even today can be obtained only at the cost of hard work. I can see two ways to make people value them, instead of contemptuously taking them for granted. One is to make them *historically conscious*, to make them *viscerally* aware of the hard way in which this state of abundance has been won. The other way is to make it *an effort* to become a full-grown member of the mature society. These are not alternatives, *both* must be exploited.

I am aware that my views on the necessity of an effort for the pupils are very unfashionable. Many thousands of teachers, especially in the United States, still believe in a permissive education in the High Schools. Let the child find out things for himself, as it were by play, and above all, do not burden his memory! How I wish that adolescent boys and girls were created for this type of education, that, like young Pascal, they could discover geometry by themselves! But even Pascal could not invent the poetry which was written before him. For us, the older generation, it is still a joy that we know so much poetry by heart. The French used to call this '*orner la mémoire*'. I am sorry for those whose memory will not be decorated, but will contain only the magazine article which they have just read and already half forgotten.

Education by play was good enough in an agricultural civilization, where the child could playfully follow the father at the plough, and his mother milking the cows. But when the father is a computer operator, and the mother is pushing buttons in her labour-saving kitchen, playful imitation will not take us far. By all means, teach mathematics with games, geography and history with films, but if you do not add to it a concentrated dose of the arts and sciences, which can be learned only with an effort, do not expect your intelligent pupils to thank you for it. I have heard enough complaints from young Americans, who went to 'modern' schools, that they had been cheated out of their right of acquiring a culture.

It is not of course surprising that the rebellious students strongly oppose views such as mine, that they want to determine their own curriculum, sit on the examination boards, or even abolish examinations altogether. What is surprising is that they are backed by so many young teachers, who ought to know better. It took the older and more responsible teachers some time to recover from the shock; their reaction is now only getting in its stride. Daniel J. Boorstin has expressed it very well: 'First . . . we must abandon the prevalent belief in the superior wisdom of the ignorant. . . . Education is learning what you didn't even know you didn't know.'* These are elementary truths. It may be a long way from this to the retreat of the protagonists of a (largely misunderstood) Deweyism, to the recognition that an education without effort is a social danger. At present everyone who dares to advocate such 'reactionary' views will be automatically accused of being in favour of the Vietnam War, of racial segregation, etc. It will not be easy to persuade those who wanted to respond to the student riots with even more permissiveness, that they were pushing the control levers in the wrong direction.

A hard apprenticeship to qualify for membership of a highly permissive, super-abundant society is a necessity for all. Competitiveness is no less important for being a necessity only for an elite. For the highly gifted and well-motivated ambitious minority a course designed for the average will be an easy game, so easy as to be boring. Such people have a *need* for obstacles to overcome, which the average man or woman would prefer to avoid. For this important minority a stable society must provide obstacle courses and ladders to climb, otherwise their energy will turn against themselves, or against society.

* *Newsweek*, 6 July 1970, p. 25.

This can be done, and it has been done successfully in the old democracies. I am convinced that a man with an overwhelming ambition towards power like Winston Churchill, had he been born in a Latin-American country, would have become a junta leader or a dictator. As it was, he kept to the rules of democracy, and though he was several times defeated in elections by non-descript opponents, he never condemned the system, and never attempted to play Coriolanus. It is very important to give such people competitive careers in which they can be socially useful, but it is equally important not to admit to these careers men or women who are power addicts, who desire power for its own sake. In democratic countries such people rarely reach the highest posts; their potential tyranny is usually discovered at an early stage of their career. After the terrible example of Stalin, one may hope that even the less safeguarded system of the USSR will be sufficient to prevent a recurrence. It would be best to exclude such people from careers which lead to power at the school-leaving age, by psychological tests. I believe that the tendency towards incipient tyranny shows itself in the character at an early age.

The mature society must offer a great diversity of ladders, in administration, the sciences, the arts, sports, entertainment, and other lines of values yet to be invented. Needless to say, it must be a *multidimensional* world of values; the one-dimensional scale of pay, already less important than it was 50 years ago, is bound to become unimportant in an age of material abundance. But let us be clear about it – however many avenues we offer towards success there is no success unless others fail. It is a distinction to be a member of a national academy only because there are so many who have not made it. The more just the method of election or promotion, the worse the fate of the unsuccessful, who cannot console themselves that they are victims of intrigues. If we wish for a world in which ambition can be rewarded by distinction, we cannot wish for a world without frustration, because distinction is a thing which cannot be democratically distributed. We cannot have excellence *and* equality.

14. THE NEW HISTORIC EDUCATION

The accumulated work of some three thousand years has created a treasure-house which is far too large for all but some very exceptional minds. C. P. Snow in his Rede Lecture (1959) on 'The Two Cultures and the Scientific Revolution' has deplored the blindness of the humanists to the wonderful achievements of science,★ the ignorance of the scientists and technologists regarding the treasures of the arts, and the almost universal blindness to the technology on which our civilization is based. Even technologists see only a small sector of it; the others take it for granted that they can get fresh water at the turn of a tap, and a television picture at the push of a button. Why should they bother their minds about it? They take notice only when the water is infected, or when the TV set fails for some reason.

How can we make the majority realize how rich they are, how much they owe to this technological civilization, which they treat with almost the same ignorance and contempt as the feudal lord treated the serfs who brought him the produce of the land of which he understood nothing? Even those very exceptional universalists who have a thirst for knowing everything, and occasionally pick up popular books or magazines on technology, have mostly only a cold, purely cerebral appreciation for it. What we need is *visceral* appreciation.

Can we make the average man proud of his heritage? I do not believe that the task is impossible, once we recognize its vital importance. First we must train the teachers and develop the technical means. It must not discourage us that the great effort in

★ See Note 11.

the USSR to make the people technologically enthusiastic, with thousands of evening lectures attended by millions of people, has brought only indifferent results, except in matters such as space travel, which have an emotional appeal even to the newspaper reader in the West. Our task is in fact more difficult, because we must make people proud and enthusiastic not for a growing technology, but for a substantially completed one. The general path which leads towards this is to put cultural history not into their heads but into their bones. I want to sketch out two educational courses, for every adolescent boy or girl, which may be able to achieve this. The first I call the *Robinson Course*, the second *Living Through History*.

THE ROBINSON COURSE

How has Man, starting with his ten fingers, made the long journey at the end of which he can produce aeroplanes, electron microscopes, millions of chemical compounds which have never existed in nature? Daniel Defoe did not dare to face the whole problem; his Robinson Crusoe had tools which were saved from the shipwreck. The numerous authors who have rewritten his tale have greatly improved it, by making him start from nothing, and bringing him up to something like the level of the crafts in the 16th century. Since that time millions of children have enjoyed this classic. On me it made an impression probably stronger than on the average child. There was, though, an even stronger influence in my life – my father, who instead of fairy tales told me stories about Edison, who, he said, had done more for mankind than all the kings taken together. But I think Robinson Crusoe also contributed to making me an inventor. When I was a student of engineering, I used to test myself before falling asleep with games such as this: 'Start with nothing in an island which has iron ore and trees, and work up to the first *lathe* with a lead-screw.'* The Robinson Course would consist of such games,

---

* This was an interesting exercise, because it made me realize that there is an *evolutionary principle* in lathes. Any lathe can make a lead-screw a little better than its own, because of the statistical equalization of the pitch in an

assisted of course not only by richly illustrated books, but also by films and practical exercises. It will not be *exactly* history. We know too little of the early inventors, often we have to substitute myths, which are usually short cuts. The real history of early inventions is full of stumblings, gropings, often of superstitions which have accidentally worked out right. The *a posteriori* short cuts may be myths to the historian, but they are more interesting for the adolescent who wants to get a comprehensive picture of technical civilization.

As I do not want to resort to pictorial illustrations, I will give only sketches of a few evolutionary lines in the Robinson Course.

Man the hunter. The club, the spear, and the first great triumph: the bow and arrow.

Man the toolmaker. Stone axes. Extracting metals from ores. Copper, bronze, iron. The first steel knife. Casting of bronze and iron. The tempering of steel, from superstition to science. The rolling mill. The first machine tools, and their evolution to modern automatic machinery.

Textiles. Spinning and hand weaving. The first loom, an astonishing example of early technological genius. The power loom, the automatic Jacquard loom. Artificial fibres. The extrusion of nylon. Mass production of nylon hosiery.

Harnessing natural forces. Water and wind. From the first steam engine to the giant turbine. From Volta's battery and Faraday's discovery of induction to the modern electric power station. Atomic power.

Transport. The horse and the oxcart. The first railway and the first motor car. The evolution of the aeroplane.

These are some of the main evolutionary lines. It would be

---

elastic nut. I learned much later that Henry Maudslay, when he made his first lathe (around 1790), utilized this principle in a most ingenious way. He made a rough lead-screw, by winding a wire on a mandrel, and cutting with a chisel between the turns. He then clamped on this a long box, filled with elder pith, which served as an elastic nut, and cut his first lead-screw with it. 150 years later Sir Thomas Merton independently realized the principle of the elastic nut, and brought it to such perfection that he could use it for the production of *optical* diffraction gratings, the best ever made until that time.

easy to multiply them. At a more advanced stage of the course instead of single lines evolutionary *trees* can be introduced, to show the transfer of know-how, first from one craft to the other, later, with the rise of applied science, the development of 'know-how sources' in academic and industrial research laboratories.

After this mainly historic, evolutionary course, a 'horizontal' view: how are the things produced which the citizen needs in his daily life; clean water, electric power, food, houses, clothing, radio and television sets, motor cars?*

Bright boys and girls will take spontaneous interest in these fascinating matters, if they are presented at an age when their natural curiosity is not yet dulled by habitual mental laziness. But it may be dry fare for the less gifted, less cerebral types. I believe that many of these can be also interested if the subject matter is presented in a manner which can *emotionally* involve them, by presenting to them not just the triumphs of technology, but also the miseries which these have relieved. There is a masterful example of this in Aldous Huxley's essay 'Hyperion to a Satyr'† on the very prosaic-looking subject of 'clean water'. I cannot do better than quote a few passages from it.

'Dirt, with all its concomitant odours and insects, was once accepted as an unalterable element in the divinely established Order of Things . . . Lotario de Conti, later Pope Innocent III, wrote a book on the *Wretchedness of Man's Condition*: . . . "dead human beings give birth to flies and worms; alive they generate worms and lice" . . . "Consider the plants, consider the trees. They bring forth flowers and leaves and fruit. But what do *you* bring forth? Nits, lice and vermin." – In the Age of Faith *Homo sapiens* was also *Homo pediculosus*.'

And so forth, in nauseating but historically truthful detail, quoting also authors much more recent than Innocent III, such

* At this point the course ought to link up with another, equally important, which introduces them to the *ecosystem*; the resources of the Earth and the biological pyramid which makes Man's existence possible. I will not enlarge on this, because there are others, far more qualified than I, who could do it better.

† In *Tomorrow and Tomorrow and Tomorrow*, a Signet Book, 1964, and also in many other editions.

as Tolstoy, who wanted everybody to be dirty in order to wipe out social distinction. But what has *homo Faber* done in the meantime? First he invented soap, then cheap soap, finally the modern detergents. These were not unmixed blessings, but *homo faber* could deal with these too, as exemplified by the Hyperion Activated Sludge Plant near Los Angeles:

'An underground river rushes into Hyperion, carrying two million gallons of water per day and a formidable quantity of muck. But happily, the ratio between muck and muckrakers remains constant. As the fecal tonnage rises, so does the population of aerobic and anaerobic bacteria. . . . First to attack the problem are the aerobes. The chemical revolution begins at a series of huge shallow pools, whose surface is perpetually foamy with the suds of Surf, Tide, Dreft and all the other monosyllables that have come to take the place of soap. . . . It has become necessary to spray the surface of the aerobes' pools with overhead sprinklers, otherwise the suds would be blown about the country-side. . . . The detergents are greedy for oxygen and prevent the aerobes from getting the air which they require. Enormous compressors must be kept working night and day to support the needs of the suffocating bacteria.

'When, with the assistance of the compressors, the aerobes have done all they are capable of doing, the sludge, now thickly concentrated, is pumped into the Digestion System . . . huge cylindrical tanks . . . in which steam pipes maintain the cherishing heat of ninety-five degrees, the temperature at which the an-aerobes are able to do their work with maximum efficiency. From something hideous and pestilential the sludge is gradually transformed by the most faithful of allies into sweetness and light . . . methane and an odourless solid which when dried, pelleted and sacked sells to the farmers at ten dollars a ton. . . . The problem of keeping a great city clean without polluting a river or fouling the beaches and without robbing the soil of its fertility has been triumphantly solved.'

We know, and the pupils in the Robinson Course must learn it too, that such a problem is never finally solved. All the better for those with any spirit left in them!

I have no illusion that even if we put an army of Aldous

Huxleys on it, with the eloquence of Madison Avenue, there would still be a hard core of pupils left, who would consider all this as 'irrelevant'. Perhaps my second suggestion can grind down this hard core to an even harder, but much smaller core.

LIVING THROUGH HISTORY

Who knows how many people, starting with Leonardo da Vinci, have dreamt of pictures which surround the viewer from all sides? I remember having this wish as a child, almost as soon as I started taking pleasure in pictures. Later I found that some science-fiction writers had perfected the dream and had visualized 'total participation machines' which make the participant see, hear and feel all the sensations of the hero. At the present stage of science the 'feelies' are beyond us, and I strongly doubt whether they will ever be possible except by tapping many nerves with microprobes. Nature has seen to it that sensations shall reach the brain only through the legitimate entrance channels – the sensory organs. But we have reached the stage at which we can supply the visual, auditory and, if required, even the olfactory organs with the sensations needed for almost total participation in a three-dimensional artificial world.

The apparatus with which this is achieved is fairly simple. Moving pictures, in colour, are taken with a stereoscopic camera, which has two extremely wide-angle, 'fisheye' lenses, spaced by the normal eye distance. The fisheye lenses can 'see' everything within a hemisphere (or even a little beyond it) and produce two strongly distorted film records, one for the right eye, one for the left. The distortion is automatically eliminated when the same camera is used as a projector; every ray of light is sent back in the direction from which it came. The problem is now to return these into the eyes of the viewer, the right picture into his right eye, the left one into his left eye. There exists a special optical screen, invented by Gabriel Lippmann (1908) which returns each ray, but spreads it out a little, vertically, so that the viewer can have his eyes a little below the projector. This, however, is difficult to make, and the viewer has only a small latitude of head movement. The simplest solution is to take any metallized reflecting screen of spherical or, more conveniently, cylindrical shape, project on it through Polaroids, and view the picture through Polaroid glasses. The three-dimensional effect is perfect, the viewer sees everything just as the camera has seen it, and he feels right in the middle of the spatial scene. This, together with stereophonic sound effects (and olfactory effects, produced by a spray), is as near as we can get to 'total participation'.*

This device could be a powerful tool of education *with emotional impact.*† I would like to see it used on young children and on adolescents, to make them *live through human history*, and remember it as they remember their own life.

Imagine that the boy or girl wakes up in the cave, with the big beasts of prey howling outside; later at the fire, with their eyes glowing in the bush. Let him feel the fear of primitive man before he started defeating them. Let him feel the pride of the prehistoric genius who invented the bow and arrow when he saw the first antelope struck down by an arrow from afar. Then let him invent agriculture and the domestication of animals, and see the first cities rising in Babylon. Let him see the Parthenon when it was new, and walk through the Forum Romanum in its ancient glory; discover America with Columbus; suffer the hardship of a medieval serf and of the worker in the time of the Industrial Revolution, and see in the end the modern Age of Affluence. (There will be no need to hide its imperfections.) If after this course he does not develop a *visceral* feeling for evolutionary ethics, if he does not feel in his bones that this hard-earned civilization is worth preserving, then, I think, he is not a man or woman but only an animal with appetites. The character-

---

* I do not want to give the impression that I am 'pushing' one of my physical inventions. It is not much of an invention. The real credit must go to the Japanese lens designers who have created such wonderful fisheye lenses as the 'Nikor'. I am not materially interested in it, nor is anybody else, and therefore it is rather unlikely that it will be launched as a commercial enterprise. A device which only one viewer can use at a time can be justified only by its unique educational value, in which I strongly believe.

† It could be of course used also for entertainment. In Note 12 I quote the horrifying vision of Ray Bradbury of the gigantic imbecility to which a device like this could lead, if it is directed towards making people mindless.

influencing drugs, which science will almost certainly put at our disposal, may be able to deal with this hard core too, but I try to believe that this hard core will be even less numerous than the one on which the Robinson Course will make no impression. I would like to make both courses, as well as the course in parenthood, compulsory also for those who leave school at 15 or 16 years of age.

This will be of course very expensive education, because the apparatus can be used on only one viewer at a time, but this ought not to be prohibitive in the Affluent Society. Mass production of educational devices which produce balanced men and women may be socially more justifiable than the mass production of motor cars.

15. THE NEW UNIVERSITY AND LIFELONG EDUCATION

A university is one of those many things which cannot be scaled up beyond modest limits. One cannot scale up a flea to the size of an elephant and expect it to be a viable animal. One comes up against laws of physics which make the monster collapse. But in scaling up universities one comes up against something even more fundamental – the simple law of logic that distinction cannot be evenly distributed, or there remains nothing of it.

Fifty years ago, and even nearer to the present date, universities were viable institutions. They took, in the industrial nations, something like 4 to 8% of an age group and educated them to become doctors, lawyers, higher administrators, scientists, engineers and teachers, with a moderate dropout.*

Here I must face the very familiar objection that the students were not the most highly gifted 4 to 8% of the population but 'the sons of the rich'. Of course there were some who had no other qualifications, and they may have been even in the majority in some Oxford colleges and (as I heard from Robert Hutchins) in the University of Virginia, before 1900. But these students seldom lined up for the final degree. They came to the university to become cultured gentlemen, or to make the right sort of friendships for life. On the whole, the moderate dropout rate at the high standard of degree examinations proved that there cannot have been too many who were merely 'sons of the rich'.

Neither were they the whole cream of the intelligence of the nation, but certainly more than a random selection. Even

* Even today the total 'wastage' in British universities is only 13·5%, and it has stood around this figure for a long time.

socialists like Lord Blackett estimate that the 5% or so admitted to British universities may have represented something like 40% of the 'cream' which can be educated to UK honours standard.* This would raise the estimate of experienced educators, such as Lord Lindsay of Birkett, or Sir John Wolfenden, who believed that only 5% of the population can profit from a university education to 12%. (It agrees well with James Bryant Conant's estimate that *at most* 15% of the population can be educated in 'hard' subjects.) This means that we can draw the lower IQ limit of those on whom a university education can 'take' at 119 (12%) instead of the more widely accepted 125 (5%). I am all the more willing to accept this, as 12% is about the fraction of educated professionals and specialists to whom a modern industrial society can offer jobs of distinction. I conclude that Britain, with the Robbins-target set at 12%, will not be in the danger zone for some time, but France with an intake of 25% of an age group, and the United States with 50%, are already well inside it.

It is not surprising that in France, where the degree standards have not been lowered, the dropout rate in 1966 (according to an OECD survey) was 72% and in the USA about 50%, with a decided tendency to rise. Much of this is of course due to women students, who do not enter the university with the intention of finishing their education, but if the standards in US colleges had not been lowered, by now the rate would be more like 80%. In both countries the student body is seething with dissatisfaction; in both the blown-up mass university is proving to be an impossibility.

Formerly the most highly gifted and motivated young men and women went to university. In spite of their talent and motivation, they had to work hard to acquire their degrees. But it was worth their while to work hard, because the university degree meant *distinction*, both social and economic. It qualified the bearer for the most respected and the best paid professions and positions. If you ask the older generation what made them work hard for their degree, they will for the most part frankly admit that it was not only the love of knowledge which drove them, but also the social and economic prospects.

* See Note 13.

The blown-up universities of the present day still imitate the old elite universities. They have the same faculties, they give the same degrees in medicine, law, economics, history, sciences, etc. (In the USA of course with some degrees in 'Home Economics' and the like thrown in.) For the most part they still claim to train their students for the same professions. In their quality some may not be far above secondary schools, but by their structure they claim to be universities.

What will be the future of the lower-grade students when they leave the universities with or without a degree? They will be *trained* for jobs, in offices, on the factory floor, or in shops, with training times from one week to a maximum of one year. Almost all jobs which they could have had without ever seeing a university.

And now we expect these young men and women with their less good brains to work hard for the love of knowledge alone, without the stick of necessity, without the carrot of success! Is it not natural that they will rather have their fun by breaking up the institutions into which they fit so badly?

Why is it that this simple argument has not become self-evident and commonplace? Because it smacks of what is called nowadays 'unashamed elitism'. Elitism is tacitly, but very efficiently, acknowledged in the USSR, where the university entrants are carefully selected for their scholastic achievements and the dropouts are sentenced to manual labour. In the great Western countries on the other hand liberals prefer to ignore the simple facts of the IQ scale and proclaim that everybody has the right to university education. For my part I am in enthusiastic agreement with the right to *higher* education, but this must not be confused with the right to attend courses which were traditionally designed for an elite in talent and motivation. The principle on which these courses were designed is very clearly expressed in the Cox Commission Report, *Crisis at Columbia*, 1969 (p. 22): 'The central educational assignment of American colleges and universities has long been to prepare functionally effective people for rather definite roles in industry, government and the established professions.'

The mismatch between this concept of the university and the

student population is already manifest. According to a survey made by *Fortune* magazine (carried out by the Yankelovich Organization, Oct. 1968) there are two fairly distinct types of student in American colleges. The 'practical ones', who by college education expect to earn more money, have a more interesting career and enjoy a better position in society, and those whom the survey calls 'forerunners', because their numbers are growing, for whom 'college means ... perhaps the opportunity to change things rather than to make out well in the existing system'.* About 58% belong to the first type, 42% to the second.

With all due respect, I cannot believe that in 1968, the year of the outbreak of the student rebellions, there were 42% sincere social reformers and revolutionaries in American colleges. I believe rather that it was the fashion to say so for those who were not of the 'practical' type. If they had been sincere they would have admitted that they went to college to have a good time before they bent their neck to the yoke. They are mismatched, dissatisfied people, who may have had their share of fun in the riots initiated by a much smaller, sincerely revolutionary minority.†

The abysmal mismatch which I have pointed out was certainly not the only cause of the student riots which broke out with such frightening intensity in 1968 and which have been smouldering since that time, with occasional outbreaks. In the United States they attached themselves to a real, idealistic cause – the sordid obscenity of the Vietnam war. But there was no Vietnam war and no Negro problem in France or in Japan and in many other countries where student riots broke out at the same time. If we look at it as a world-wide phenomenon we can observe only two causes common to all countries. (1) The age-group of 18 to 25 is highly inflammable and it has its last fling at revolt at this age, before they have to bend their shoulders to the responsibilities of the job and the family, and (2) universities are *soft* institutions, meant to instruct young people who come to them for knowledge, not to break them in. These causes were active also in

* *Youth in Turmoil*, Time-Life International, 1969, p. 32.

† See Note 14.

countries where the universities are still essentially elitist, such as Japan.* But in the countries in which university education has been extended far beyond the ranks of the elite, the mismatch is sufficient by itself to make the mass-university an impossibility.

In a mature, rich society everybody must have the right to higher education, but the mismatch, bad enough at present, will become unbearable. Let me repeat, the mismatch now exists between the poor *IQ-Motivation* index of the majority on the one hand, and the conception of the university which prepares its students for elite jobs on the other. The mature society will not have very many more professions and positions of distinction to offer than are available at present. We must not attempt the impossible and try to educate the majority for non-existent jobs. We must educate them to be happy, balanced, cultured men and women.

The specialist universities may take 10 to 15% of the population, which appears to be a reasonable match between talents and higher professions. But the mass university, which takes the rest, must be an *extension of high school and an introduction to life-long learning*. Rather than copy the MIT, Harvard, Cambridge or the Sorbonne, these ought to be on the lines of old Oxford, or of the old University of Virginia, and educate cultured gentlemen and gentlewomen.

What I advocate is not new, it is only very unfashionable. It is the revival or continuation of the 'General Education Movement' in American universities† which was powerfully initiated by Robert Hutchins in the University of Chicago, starting in 1929; but after he left, in 1951, the university reverted to the standard specialist pattern, with PhDs taking precedence over

---

* The malaise in civilization which manifests itself in student revolts shows itself in the purest form in Japan, where their slogan is *funsai*: pulverize! There is not the slightest trace of a constructive element in it, only a hatred of the establishment, of the industrial order, and of course of the United States. Some older observers, such as Edward Seidensticker ('The Pulverisers', Letter from Tokyo, *Encounter*, June 1970) recognize in it with a shudder a new incarnation of the murderous irrationality which broke out in the thirties, and drove Japan with firmly closed eyes into the World War.

† See Christopher Jencks and David Riesman, *The Academic Revolution*, Doubleday, New York, 1968.

general culture. In spite of much goodwill, the American universities and colleges have conspicuously failed to give a taste for knowledge to the less gifted and less motivated students. Respect for culture is much lower in the States than in many of the much poorer countries, especially in the communist countries.

Whether the mass university will give degrees or not is irrelevant. A degree shared by, say, 70% of the population cannot be of much importance. But it must give an appreciation of civilization to all, and a love of knowledge and of the arts, with a disposition to improve it during the rest of their lives to as many as possible. I would not hold out much hope of achieving this through an education, however well designed, unless the students come already well prepared for it by courses, such as were outlined in the last two chapters, in their more impressionable years. Except for a (not unimportant) minority who undergo a mental change around that age, the character is fully formed at 18, and it is too late for the acquisition of new attitudes.

Institutions do not like to be demoted, so let us call the mass university the 'new university' and the elite institutions 'specialized universities'. I think that the new university course ought not to extend beyond two or at most three years. After that, it ought to send all those who have an inclination for it on a 'wandering year' in a foreign country, having duly prepared them with language courses. The exchange of not only hundreds of thousands but millions of young men and women is an enormous social-economic problem, but it must be faced, because it may be a great contribution to world peace, second only to the establishment of a world state. A large-scale exchange of youth with the developing countries is particularly desirable, also particularly difficult. It is easiest between advanced countries with a common language. At any time there are at least 100,000 young Australians living in England, where they spend one to three years. There also exists a spontaneous stream of young Americans towards other countries, but a part of this is not a healthy phenomenon. The hippie colony in Crete, living in caves, infected by hepatitis, or the mendicant hippies from Florence to Katmandu, are pathological symptoms. I do not wish them to be stopped by force, but by an education and an organization of society which would produce less misfits.

I have emphasized that a permissive society requires a hard apprenticeship which teaches boys and girls to make efforts, intellectual and ethical. But this belongs in the formative years, the earlier the better. The permissive society starts at the university. What I advocate is almost the exact opposite of what happens at present with young Americans, who after an extremely permissive school enter a very exacting university, such as the MIT or Harvard. Such a system can work only with an elite, who, in most cases, from the influence of their family, or by natural aptitude, have the ambition to work hard and to acquire knowledge. For the great majority, 'without the carrot of distinction', the university must be made an attractive place.

Training for jobs will not be the 'central educational assignment' of the new university, because we can expect that the very diversified jobs which an advanced mature society will offer to all except the 10 to 15% professional elite will be at least as easily learned *on the job* as they are today. Exceptions may be the artistic crafts, because they are hobbies as well as professions. Nowadays doctors in the US often send their ageing patients to 'hobby consultants', so that after their retirement they shall be able to fix their interest and their energies on some subject which will save them from helpless boredom. Let us face the disagreeable prospect – in a technologically highly advanced mature society, young people at 20 may be in a similar position to that confronting those of 60 today. *Nobody ought to leave the new university without having found at least one lifelong interest.*

I wrote many years ago that 'work which is no longer necessary to sustain life will have to be retained as *occupational therapy*'. The 'do-it-yourself' movement, the hobbies which imitate work, are indeed little other than occupational therapy if their purpose is only to save people from boredom. But we must not be satisfied with mental balance if it is just the absence of boredom, just as physical health is much more than the absence of illness. An activity performed with the subjective feeling of freedom, without constraints, is an enrichment of life, and richness is also more than the absence of poverty.

It ought to be incomparably easier to enrich the life of young people in a diversified mature society, than to enrich that of the people around 60, who have to give up their daily drug of hard work and for whom the doctor prescribes 'hobbies'. The young have their choice of all the pleasures and treasures of love and family, sports, play, the arts and sciences. After early years in a loving family, after a primary and high school which has made them appreciate their luck in being born into such a rich society, there cannot be many left who are misfits in every one of these, and want to get kicks out of drugs, crime or revolt.

The new university must be an attractive and agreeable place, to which the citizen will wish to return for shorter or longer sabbaticals in his mature age. Immerse them in good music, make them familiar with the visual art of all ages, prepare them for the travels which they will soon undertake in all parts of the world. All this will be offered to the young people, but not quite free. The social responsibility, which has already been inculcated into them by their earlier schools, must be reinforced, and they must be made ready to give, as well as to receive. I believe that if it is to be a world worth living in, people must be at least as willing to give personal service as they are now willing to go into dull production jobs. Would it be too difficult to make them understand that a smiling waiter or shop-assistant fills as honourable and useful a place in society as the girl who sits at a punching machine in a factory? Everybody, except those in the specialized professions (which are also services), must be prepared to take his turn in a service job, at least at one period in his or her life.

Perhaps the most important task of the new university is to prepare all who are capable for it to lifelong education. The high ideal is what Werner Jaeger has called '*paideia*'. I cannot do better than describe it in the beautiful words of Lewis Mumford:*

'*Paideia* is education looked upon as a life-long transformation of the human personality, in which every aspect of life plays a part. Unlike education in the traditional sense, *paideia* does not limit itself to the conscious learning process, or to introducing the young into the social heritage of the community. *Paideia* is

---

* Lewis Mumford, *The Transformations of Man*, Allen & Unwin, London, 1957, p. 187.

rather a task of giving force to the act of living itself: treating every occasion in life as a means of self-fabrication, and as parts of the converting facts into values, processes into purposes, hopes and plans into consummations and realizations. *Paideia* is not merely a learning: it is making and shaping a man himself as the work of art that *paideia* seeks to form.'

This is a very lofty ideal. Perhaps Goethe was the man who realized it most perfectly in his wonderful, lifelong maturation. But though very few may be able to scale the full height, many more can find a worthwhile, meaningful life on the lower slopes.

16.   STABILITY

The minimum requirement for a stable society is that it shall not run into catastrophes. But by their very nature, catastrophes develop suddenly out of states which one may consider as not far from 'normal'.* If we want to be safe, we must watch carefully for even small signs of economic distress or difficulty of psychological adaptation and make sure that the countervailing forces start acting in good time.

The stability of a dynamic system is a scientific concept which in recent decades has become one of the central problems of engineering research. The popular conception of it is still rather primitive. The word 'stability' evokes the school example of a ball on a concave dish, which will return to the lowest point every time it is pushed out of it. The opposite to this is the unstable position of a ball on the top of a hill, which must roll off at the slightest displacement.

This picture is not satisfactory, because our social system is not static; it undergoes continual change. A simple model of a changing but stable social system is the progress of a car, driving through a valley. It need not be a motor car, bound to run on a highway, it can be a jeep. The increasing steepness of the mountain-side will drive it back towards the trough. But this would be a far too optimistic picture of things as they are. We are rather driving along a mountain ridge, with gentle slopes at both sides, but leading right and left to precipices where there is no stopping. When the driver has for a time allowed the vehicle to find its way

* Moreover, the increasing complication of the modern state and the destructive potential of science make it easier for small groups of mentally unstable individuals to initiate processes with frightful consequences. See Note 15.

by itself, his best chance may be pulling back with a jerk when the precipice is approaching. This is more or less how we are managing our economy. Can we not do better?

Some years ago physicists discovered a surprising method for stabilizing a vehicle on a ridge. Let the mountain ridge be see-sawing around its crest as fulcrum; right side up, left side down, and then the reverse. It can then be shown that if the amplitude of this oscillation and its frequency are high enough, the car will always return to the ridge. It will never come to a rest, but it will never fall into the precipice. It may be a disagreeable ride, but perfectly safe.*

This case of dynamic stability, like many others discovered by science, is clearly contra-intuitive. There are more familiar examples. A juggler who balances a billiard ball on the tip of a cue makes use of a similar principle. Nobody can balance a ball on a steady point, but it can be done if the cue performs a gentle rotation, thus converting the problem into one of dynamic stability.

A more general and powerful method for stabilizing an intrinsically unstable system is *feedback*. This means observing the system, and when it shows signs of deviating from the desired state, applying a restoring force *at the right time*. The emphasis is on the 'right time', because when the deviation is noticed it may be too late. *Every control device must be a predictor.*

This can be explained in the simple example of a pendulum, which we want to swing between two limits. Let it get an unforeseen impulse, for instance from the wind, so that it tends to overshoot the limit. If we put a rigid stop at the limit, the excess momentum will be reversed and the pendulum will try to overshoot the opposite stop, so this is not a good method. It would evidently be better to extract the excess kinetic energy of the pendulum before it has reached the limit.

The pendulum is a simple system because it has only one period:

---

* This is a mechanical illustration of a principle for stabilizing charged particles in an electrostatic field, discovered in 1959 by Ralph Wuerker and his associates in the TRW Laboratories. See Note 16. It is not quite a precise illustration, because the vehicle ought to be prevented from being thrown up in the air.

acting on it a quarter cycle before its maximum excursion ensures fair control. If the Stock Exchange were so simple, the central banks would have long learned the trick of raising the bank-rate before the stocks and shares rose to an unhealthy peak. In fact prediction of stock prices, even for short times, is a very difficult matter, and the central banks usually react too late, causing a violent collapse.

The Stock Exchange is a particularly complicated system, because its intrinsic instability has its roots in a human phenomenon, without a counterpart in nature – *anticipation*. Everybody who plays the Stock Exchange has a model of its expected behaviour in his mind, everyone is trying to guess the expectations of the majority, which will determine the rise or fall of the shares. Anticipation is also the base of the capitalistic system; but subscribers are supposed to form their expectations of the soundness of a new enterprise on expert opinion rather than on the general trend of the stock market. There is an element of gambling in this too, but much less than in the attitude of the speculator. J. M. Keynes, though himself a great gambler, thought at one time that nothing would counteract the instability of the Stock Exchange short of making the acquisition of shares 'an indissoluble bond, like marriage'. Later he conceded a possibility of divorce: one cannot expect the shareholder to live all his life on dividends, he must be able to sell, but there must be conditions restricting sale. If we are to achieve economic stability the Stock Exchange must become less of a 'casino', as Keynes called it. Gambling is an expression of the very widespread but anti-social human dream of getting rich without work. It is so deep-rooted that not even the communist countries have dared to suppress it; they have directed it into the less harmful channels of state lotteries and premium bonds. It must be possible to separate it also in the free economies from the very justifiable process of exchanging 'deferred gratification' for a share in new productive enterprises. In Chapter 11 I advocated the financing of as much as possible of the public sector by private savings, through a new type of bonds. Such bonds will most easily be acceptable as investments when speculation is restricted, for instance by restrictive conditions on 'divorce'.

Another instability in our system, of which we have become painfully aware in recent years, is the mechanism of 'cost-push' inflation. The trades unions present their wage claims one after the other; the highest rise obtained at once becomes the norm. The anticipation of inflation makes it certain that inflation will continue. The manufacturers also raise their prices one after the other, in a leapfrogging procession. There appears no other way of stopping this process than by *tying the demands together*. Let the unions thrash out their wage claims between themselves, and present them *in toto* to the employer, with the State as arbitrator.* Tying wages to the cost of living is of no use so long as there is no limit to their rising together. Tying them to production is a sound principle when applied to the whole economy, but it becomes unsound when it is applied to single production units. It is not the merit of the wage earner if his productivity has been increased by heavy capital investment, nor is it the fault of others if they have lagged behind in other units, where there was no technological change. In brief, the only remedy which is likely to help is the same which the engineer applies when motors which ought to pull together fall out of step; he applies a stabilizing constraint by tying them together. This remedy has been obvious for a long time to economists such as Beveridge, but it is seldom advocated, partly because it seems hopeless in the face of the determined resistance of the trades unions, partly perhaps also because it appears too great an obstacle to free competition. I do not think that this fear is justified. Wages are already being equalized between competing manufacturers, but by a one-after-the-other process, which has an escalating tendency. Is there much to lose, is there not much more to gain, if wage adjustments happen simultaneously?

In the past large disturbances in the economic system were terminated, if at all, by bankruptcies, unemployment and the resignation which these brought with them. The great crash of the thirties was terminated only by the war. Compared with the thirties we are now living in a Golden Age. We have realized that an economic disturbance is not a natural catastrophe, it is caused by human agencies, and we can do something about them.

* See Note 17.

If unemployment on anything like the scale of the thirties were threatening (when the *smallest* figure in Britain was 10 per cent!) governments would rather face runaway inflation than a revolution. But we are still far from being able to solve, without hardship to at least some classes, the four conditions of a stable national economy:

> Full employment
> Steady growth
> Balance of foreign payments
> Stable prices.

It was the last condition which was and is violated, even in the most successful countries, such as Germany and Japan, chiefly because it hits the class which is least able to hit back – the pensioners while favouring the debtors.

There can be little doubt that the next step towards improved stability will require increased state intervention. The 'free-for-all' fight for wages and profits must be regulated. The question is only to what extent, and at what price? I cannot see in the 'free-for-all' any praiseworthy manifestation of personal freedom. Is the right of comparatively small unions to throw big spanners in the machinery by strikes, or the right of some manufacturers to disturb the equilibrium by price increases, so sacred? On the contrary, I think that creative private initiative has been badly obstructed in the last few years, and the initiative of the State for introducing long-term reforms even more. But the fear that a clumsy intervention by the State could also damage worthwhile liberties is not quite unfounded.

This is where I believe that science will help. The social-economic system with its thousands of interdependent units, connected by immensely numerous and complicated relationships, has grown above our head. No human brain can grasp it all, even less predict its development in the future. We grab at the controls one after the other, and the effect is either almost nothing, or even contrary to what was intended. I believe that the electronic computer has come just in time to help out where the human mind fails. Of this I will have more to say in a later chapter.

17. FREEDOM IN A MATURE SOCIETY

How much freedom can we preserve in a mature society? If we want to give a reasonable answer to this question, we cannot avoid analysing this value, which has given rise to more confusion than perhaps any other social idea. On the face of it, freedom appears to be a perennial value. I know of no society in which 'a free man' did not have a laudatory connotation.* (Though curiously the near-synonym 'liberal' has become a byword in certain American circles.) But this universal lip-service makes one suspect that the idea behind the word must have undergone protean changes. Remember that the revivalist meetings of Hitler used to end with the shout '*Herr, mach uns frei!*', 'Lord, set us free!'

The basic distinctions 'freedom from' and 'freedom for' can equally well be used for clarifying the subject as for sophistic confusion. '*Freedom from fear*' and '*freedom from want*' use the term 'freedom' only as a negative. They could be equally well expressed positively by the slogan '*security and comfort*', though, curiously, they would lose much of their appeal. '*Freedom from exploitation*', the great socialist slogan, is somewhat less simple. It means that each man shall be fully rewarded for his *own* work, and what this is has become rather difficult to decide in the case of a man manipulating an automated blast furnace or petrol refinery with pushbuttons. One can express

---

* I can remember only one condemnation. The Commissar Tibor Szamuely, in the short-lived Hungarian Commune of 1919, declared that 'freedom is a bourgeois ideology'. A hideous thought, expressed in an appropriately hideous jargon.

it positively by the rather vague wish for 'social justice'.

The 'freedoms for' take us nearer to the psychological meaning of freedom. The 'freedoms from' are services which a perfect social organization ought to provide. The 'freedoms for' relate to domains in which the citizen ought to be left alone to make his choice and to follow his own will. It is these freedoms which, many people fear, will be threatened in well-organized societies of the future. This fear, expressed in innumerable dystopias,* is not quite unfounded. There is a basic conflict between individual will and the requirements of an organized society. Only compromise solutions are possible, of which I shall have more to say later.

'Free will' was long a stumbling block for philosophers; it has become much clearer to our modern scientific view. The old attitude was naïvely expressed in Laplace's determinism. Once the initial state of every atom in the world is determined, the world runs down like clockwork. Hence, as the present state of the world is determined, it is determined for all time.

To the modern scientist this is on a level with the oriental belief in 'Kismet'. The fate of everybody is written – but in a book to which nobody has access! For the scientist a book to which nobody has access does not exist. Neither does 'the present state' of the universe exist, because by the 'Uncertainty Principle' we could not determine it without altering it. But it is not necessary to go down to fundamentals in order to find a niche for human free will. I am free in my decisions so long as I am *ignorant* of the state of the myriad variables in my mind which may have long predetermined my decision.

For minds with a literary or historical background, an equation of free will with partial ignorance will appear highly unpalatable. Freedom is a value, ignorance is not. For the scientific mind there is nothing shocking in this; why should the mind of man not

---

* Perhaps the first who expressed this fear was Yevgeny Zamyatin, in his nightmare novel *WE*, written in 1924. Men and women are made into perfect, happy robots by a little operation: 'The location of the Centre of Fantasy is the latest discovery of science in The One State. This Centre is a miserable little cerebral node in the region of the Bridge of Varioli. A triple cauterization of this node with X-rays, and you are cured of Fantasy.'

locate his values in the domains in which he is ignorant (not independent) of necessity?

Philosophers have continually been aware of the conflict between this fundamental tendency of the human mind and social necessity, and this is probably what makes the history of freedom and free will one of the least satisfactory chapters of philosophy. From Aristotle to Hegel, few philosophers could abstain from preaching a sermon and from giving ethical directives instead of analysis. Hegel's definition 'freedom is the recognition of necessity' is a particularly transparent example.* Against such sermonizing David Hume objected: 'There is no method of reasoning more common, and yet none more blameable, than, in philosophical disputes, to endeavour the refutation of any hypothesis, by a pretence of its dangerous consequences to religion and morality.'† But the old philosophers were really in a grave dilemma. Freedom had to be constrained to willing the right thing. Free will, the choice between good and evil, had to be admitted, otherwise how could the criminal be punished? How could he be blamed if he could do nothing else? And if he could do nothing else, how could the Deity who created him be absolved from his sin? Hume, with his unique commonsense, simply refused to dive into this 'ocean of doubt, uncertainty and contradiction'.

For us there is no need to dive into this philosophical morass. Society must be protected against the 'free will' of the criminal or else it will not be able to provide 'freedom from fear' for the majority. But the definition of anti-social acts is a delicate balance between the rights of the individual and the stability of society. It can only too easily shift towards totalitarianism; a logical consequence of the Hegelian view of freedom.

'Free' choice, that is to say ignorance about the inner constraints which determine the choice, is a necessary condition of freedom, but it does not become complete until we add to it a *valuation* of choices. Hobbes and Locke have rightly emphasized that man's liberty is not so much the freedom of his will in choos-

---

* More completely: 'Freedom is nothing but the recognition and adoption of such universal objects as Right and Law.'

† David Hume, *Concerning Human Understanding*, Section VIII, 'On Liberty and Necessity', Pt. II.

ing, but the freedom of *doing what he wills*, without constraint or impediment. This is the real dilemma, because the space of desires cannot exactly coincide with the space of possible and permissible actions. The Pleasure Principle must conflict with the Reality Principle. At best we can work for a good compromise, on the one hand a permissive society, on the other an education which restricts anti-social desires. It does not appear possible to construct a new 'utilitarian calculus' which weighs one against the other. Only somewhat risky social experiments can show whether, for instance, a relaxation of sexual repression leads to bearable or unbearable social consequences. Later on I will discuss some hopeful ways of taking the risk out of social experiments by *simulation*, but for the time being one must admit that there is nothing more difficult to quantify than man's urges.

There is however one aspect of freedom which is amenable to measurement. This is the statistical, *a posteriori* freedom; a concept introduced some years ago by my brother André Gabor and myself.* We do not ask about the desires of individuals, but about the use which they have actually made of existing choices. The freedom is measured by the spread or *diversity* of the choices of a population, with the qualification that this diversity must not be imposed by constraints. Take as an example freedom in male dress. The uniforms of soldiers are far more diverse than the dresses of civilians, but this diversity is imposed by the organization; the soldier has no choice whatever in his dress. On the other hand there exists no rule which forbids a bank employee to wear a boiler suit: if nevertheless we find bank employees fairly uniformly dressed, we conclude that this freedom in fact does not exist. Or take the freedom to vote for your party in a democracy: if we find that the lowest income brackets have voted communist, those a little higher socialist, and in the highest conservative, was there any real freedom? We conclude that there was no real freedom, because the vote was determined by income, and income is not a matter of free choice. Of course we do not dispute that even this represents a degree of freedom over a country where there is only one party, because it is undoubtedly a freedom for a *class* to express its discontent.

* See Note 18.

Statistical *post facto* freedom may be a valuable social indicator, chiefly for showing up hidden constraints, once sufficient statistical material is available. At present such material is very scarce, but we have been able to obtain some interesting results. There are Swedish statistics which list the IQ of the subject, his profession and the profession of his father. The investigation shows that the IQ of the son so strongly determines his social status that adding the status of the father as a second factor only makes a very small difference. We conclude that social mobility in Sweden has reached a high degree of perfection. Though the IQ may be an accident of birth, just as much as the status of one's father, this is not a restriction of freedom, because by the tenets of our civilization we do not regard the dependence of profession on the IQ as an undesirable constraint. This was different in the Middle Ages, when the privilege of birth was unquestioned. It may be different again in a future society which has learned to control intelligence artificially. We may then hear the slogan: 'Equal IQ for all!'

The last example shows that the call for freedom arises only when a constraint becomes *avoidable*. Until then it remains a matter of divine justice (or injustice); when it becomes avoidable it is a matter for social justice, and at once breeds new conflicts. The progress of science is producing examples all the time. For instance, not so very long ago people with diseased kidneys had to die, now a few can have their life prolonged by grafts, and many more by kidney machines – but still not all! In this case the duty of society is clear, but there are others in which the progress of science creates very questionable new freedoms. Experts seem to agree that the predetermination of the sex of infants is not many years away. It will then be up to parents to decide what until now was left to Nature. Will they spontaneously maintain the equilibrium of the sexes? If yes, they will have freedom only in the sense of Hegel's dictum 'freedom is the recognition of necessity'. If no, the State may have to intervene and impose what will appear as a new hardship.

One can say, very generally, that the progress of scientific civilization withdraws more and more domains from the jurisdiction of Nature and makes them subjects of conscious human decision. With one hand science enlarges our freedom, with the other it gives rise to new human conflicts.

The increasing complexity of industrial society on a crowded Earth has a similar but rather worse effect. It extends freedom from want, but at the same time it restricts many 'freedoms for' which we have grown accustomed to. I give below a short list of 'freedoms for', of individuals and groups, which have now become questionable. I have put asterisks to those freedoms which we take for granted in our liberal-democratic societies, but which were punishable (often by death) in the past, and are still punished in some countries.*

FREEDOMS OF THE INDIVIDUAL

* He or she can take early to smoking, drink or sex, without any other consequences than disapproval by parents or teachers. He or she will fall foul of the law only when taking to marijuana or hard drugs.

* After the age of consent he can marry whomever he likes, regardless of heredity, and in some countries he can also make a permanent liaison with a person of his own sex, so long as he does not seduce minors.

GROUP FREEDOMS

The family has the right to educate the child well or badly. The welfare services and private organizations will intervene only in cases of gross cruelty. It receives encouragement to produce more children.

* *Trade unions* in some countries can break written agreements without any legal consequences.

* *Groups of workers* can start unofficial strikes, disrupting the economy and laying off many more than their own number, without being answerable for the damage caused.

* *Political parties* in some countries can make it their declared aim to break down the established system.

* An interesting list of crimes which were formerly punishable, often by death, and which we do not consider as such may be found in Pitirim A. Sorokin's *Social and Cultural Dynamics*, Vol. 2, 'Fluctuations of Systems of Truth, Ethics and Law', The Bedminster Press, New York, 1962, pp. 530–3.

* *Groups of students*, even if they are in a minority, can obstruct college or university education or damage university property, with the maximum consequence of expulsion for a limited time.
* *The press* is free to print the memoirs of criminals and other matter on the borderline of 'intended to deprave and corrupt'.

The mass media are free to fill much of their time with scenes of violence.

Industrial enterprises are free to manufacture and to push by all methods of advertising goods whose effect will be anti-social in the long run, such as (to mention only a mild example) 'throw-away' containers, which will swell the mass of solid waste, and pollute the air when they are incinerated. They are also free to dismiss redundant employees, with certain provisions of sever-ance pay, but without any obligation to find them new jobs.

The State in its relation with other states can act as an immoral being, for instance it can supply arms to countries without any responsibility for what they will do with the arms.

Every one of these freedoms conflicts at some point with the freedom of others. We must tolerate a certain amount of conflict, because this is the price we must pay for a free society. It is sheer hypocrisy to believe that people could be made satisfied with *feeling* free to do certain acts, and yet voluntarily refrain from doing them, in the interests of society. Actualized freedom *is* disorder, which means not only diversity but also conflict. The continual conflict and strife in a free society provides the *excitement* which is a necessity for Irrational Man.* It may well be that our liberal-democratic society has overreached itself in some of its freedoms, but we must be very careful with restrictions in favour of a dull order, which might make the need for excitement break out in even more irrational and damaging channels.

* Institutions must not be too perfect, because man is far from perfect. A distinguished industrial psychologist wrote, long ago: 'To certain characters the joy of having a grievance is incalculable.' (Miss May Smith, 'General Psychological Problems Confronting an Investigator', *4th Annual Report of the Industrial Fatigue Research Board*, London, 1924.) Two generations of personnel managers have echoed her feelings. It would be unfair to deprive these characters of their grievances, but we need not worry – we can never achieve it!

18.   THE ART OF PREDICTION

The governments of the near future, if they are to serve us well, will have immensely difficult problems to solve. They will have to steer the world towards a stable ecosystem, in which we do not exhaust natural resources faster than they are replaced or substitutes found. They will have to engineer the great transformation from the whirling-dervish economy of the epoch of exponential growth towards a mature society, first in the highly industrialized countries, later in the rest of the world. They will have to devise an education which replaces the pressure of the economics of scarcity by personal responsibility. And all this with as little *dirigisme* as possible, maintaining all the time the maximum of freedom which is compatible with social stability.

'*Gouverner c'est prévoir*' was never more true than now, nor was it ever more difficult. The rulers of the past had little other than past history and their instincts to guide them, but in a much slower developing world historical parallels were still of some use. Today we must look farther ahead, and surprises which make long-term planning difficult are happening with alarming frequency.*

Where can the rulers take their wisdom? I do not underrate the ethical component of wisdom. Who could doubt that we would live in a better and safer world if the leaders of the super-powers were men with the moral stature of an Albert Schweitzer or a William Penn? But even given the best will, there will be

---

* We have come a long time since the nineties, when an old statesman revealed to the young Winston Churchill the wisdom of a long life: 'Nothing ever happens!'

difficult technical operational problems to solve and where can one turn for advice if not to science?

Until fairly recently, science was very badly prepared for dealing with systems as complicated as a country, let alone the whole globe, in which everything is connected with everything by world-wide instantaneous communications, and interwoven, but often conflicting, interests. Such systems produce the phenomenon of *collective interactions*, for instance coalitions and mental epidemics. It is just in this field that science has suffered its most conspicuous defeat, when in the development of controlled fusion devices it first encountered collective interactions on a grand scale. Science has long ago dealt successfully with ordinary gases, in which a collision involves only two molecules. But in the high-temperature, energy-charged plasma of fusion devices all ions are connected with one another by long-range forces, and collectively they develop configurations (one could also call them conspiracies), so organized that great numbers of ions can break *together* out of magnetic bottles which would retain even the most energetic ones if they tried to escape singly. This is because in the plasma every ion, as it were, 'knows' of every other ion, by long-range forces. But what is the complication of the plasma compared with that of human societies, in which individuals and groups not only know what the others are doing, but are *trying to anticipate what they will be doing*! We have seen examples of this in the case of the Stock Exchange, where everybody is trying to anticipate whether the others will be buying or selling and in the much more dangerous case of the arms race of the great powers, who are trying to anticipate the next weapons system of the other. Man, like all the higher animals, is an anticipator, otherwise he would not have survived. Now, in a closely-coupled world, overcharged with energy, the game of anticipations is threatening us with destruction – unless we refine the art of prediction so as to give the controllers superior powers of anticipation.

Not only the unaided human mind, but the intellect aided by the methods of mathematical analysis, such as have been developed by the great mathematicians of the last 300 years, is unable to cope with the type of complications presented by social-economic problems. The situation would be almost hopeless, were it not that the electronic computer was invented, just in time.

The electronic computer is completely stupid, even more so than the arithmetic child prodigies who can multiply in their heads numbers with five or more digits, without being able to say how they do it. But it has an almost unlimited capacity for imitation, or, to use the scientific terms, for 'modelling' or 'simulation'. Most of our thinking is done with mental models. The bridge player has a model in his head of the habits of his partner and opponents, the industrialist of his firm, of his competitors and of the market. These models are wonderful in their variety, but less so in precision and extension, and even less in their predicting powers.

I derive most of my confidence in the computer simulation of economic and social systems from the pioneering work of Professor Jay W. Forrester at MIT.* In Forrester's own words: 'Our social systems belong to the class called multi-loop nonlinear feedback systems. In the long history of evolution it has not been necessary for man to understand these systems until very recent historical times. Evolutionary processes have not given us the mental skill needed to properly interpret the dynamic behavior of the systems of which we have now become a part.'

This, I believe, will hardly be disputed. Everybody knows how unsuccessful governments and their economic advisers have been in stopping inflation, and how often their actions produced results opposite to those intended. But it is a long step from this admission to the stage of trusting the computer, which is admittedly a mindless device and must be fed by human intelligence. The encouragement comes from Forrester's observation: the human mind is capable of specifying the components of even very complicated economic systems, and even the relationship between any two of them, *bit by bit*, but it cannot embrace the whole simultaneously, and it fails even more conspicuously in predicting the dynamic behaviour of such a system. On the other hand the computer, once it has been given a *complete* specification of the

* Jay W. Forrester, *Industrial Dynamics*, MIT Press, Cambridge, Mass., 1961; *Principles of Systems*, Wright-Allen Press, Cambridge, Mass., 1968; *Urban Dynamics*, MIT Press, Cambridge, Mass., 1969; *World Dynamics*, Wright-Allen Press, Cambridge, Mass., 1971.

system, however complicated, can trace its dynamic consequences with perfect reliability.

Forrester and his collaborators were led to this contention not by any *a priori* reasoning, but by many years of observation and experience with problems of increasing complication. They first started with Industrial Dynamics, when they were called in as consultants by industrial firms in difficulties, who had found that events had turned out contrary to expectations. They fed into the machine the data supplied by the corporations, with their policies. It then turned out that the computer model gave not the expected but the *actually experienced* history of the firm. This means that the model was correct, only its dynamic behaviour was quite different from what was intended, because it was 'contra-intuitive'. Often, when the bad luck was blamed on surprises of the market, or unexpected moves by the competitors, it was found to have been caused by the well-intentioned policies of the corporation itself.

The next step was Urban Dynamics; the dynamics of industrial cities. This began in February 1968, when John D. Collins, former Mayor of Boston, joined MIT as Professor of Urban Affairs, and brought with him a wealth of experience on the contra-intuitive behaviour of townships. Forrester and his group constructed a computer model, which could make a run, correspond-ing to some 200 years of city history in a few minutes. One could therefore rapidly test on it a very great number of policies. Generally the industrial town, starting from a green field or a village, first grows rapidly, and then after a time the difficulties start. It decays or, at best, stagnates. This is the time when creative policies are called for. The results were striking. *Every policy which brought an improvement in the short run led in the long run to a state worse than before.* Only unpopular policies helped, with some hardship at the start, such as demolishing 10% of low-cost housing every year.

Such striking and unpleasant conclusions could not of course fail to evoke much adverse criticism. The results were blamed on Forrester's 'arbitrary' assumptions. But Forrester could point out that these results were to a high extent insensitive to the details of the assumed laws of interrelations. For instance, so long as low-cost housing and assistance exercised *some* attraction on unskilled or underemployed people from other towns, it remains the right policy to demolish a part of it every year.

The next step, World Dynamics, was a bold one. At the request of the Club of Rome, Professor Forrester undertook the modelling of a world-wide economic system. (The Club of Rome is a small international body of people interested in the future, convened by the eminent Italian industrialist Dr Aurelio Peccei.)* This computer model, of which a brief sketch is given in Note 19, is of impressive complication, far beyond the capacity of any human mind. Even so a computer run from the year 1900 to AD 2100 takes only a few minutes.

The results are again striking, one could even say dramatic. Almost every run leads to a catastrophe in well under 100 years, by exhaustion of natural resources coupled with increasing pollution caused by industrial expansion. Almost any attempt to boost the quality of life beyond its present level speeds up the catastrophe. The runs which lead to a stable ecosystem are again strongly contra-intuitive and unpopular. One of these pre-supposes, in 1970, a reduction of the capital investment rate by 40%, of the birthrate by 50%, natural resource usage rate by 75%, of food production by 20%. The level at which world population stabilizes is about three thousand million, somewhat less than the present.

These results will of course evoke even stronger criticism than Urban Dynamics. The assumption regarding pollution will probably be considered as too pessimistic. Also, complicated as the model is, it does not do justice to the complication of the world system. One ought to expect at least a division into developed and underdeveloped, or, better, into free-market, communist and underdeveloped countries. This would be too much to expect of a model which has been put together in a few months. It can be considered only as an 'admonitory tale', but with much more weight than the admonitory tales of science fiction. It is a forerunner of many more models which, it may be hoped, will soon be constructed under an international programme.†

* See Aurelio Peccei, *The Chasm Ahead*, Macmillan, London, 1969.

† At the time of writing the work is being continued and the computer programme perfected by Professor Dennis Meadows, MIT.

With all these reservations, I think that we must take the warning contained in the dramatic results of this forerunner very seriously; certainly to the point of encouraging the development of its more perfect successors with the trifling sums of money which it will require. (Trifling not only in comparison to the potential importance of the results, but also compared to the cost of other international organisations.) But we must do more than that. These computer simulations, originated mostly by engineers and applied mathematicians, will probably evoke hostile reactions from economists and social scientists, who might regard these newcomers as amateurish bunglers. This would be a grave mistake. Instead of unhelpful scepticism they ought to offer collaboration. Computer simulations require not only every scrap of factual knowledge which we can put into them, but also intuition, in particular when the human factors will appear in them. But instead of trying to understand and predict the whole system intuitively, which is patently impossible, intuition must be applied *piecemeal*. Leave the complication to the computer, it will do the rest better than any human mind or even an academy of social scientists could do it. Let computers contend with computers!

Let me now assume, provisionally, that some consensus of computers will come about, and that they confirm that we are running into some sort of catastrophe unless we mend our ways radically. This would open a new chapter in human history and a new ethic; responsibility for a hundred years or more ahead. It is not quite new; our ancestors built palaces and houses to last for hundreds of years, and planted oak trees which would give shadow only to the third generation. We have lost this spirit only in the last hundred years of growth addiction, with irresponsible depletion of the resources of the Earth, with increasing pollution and with the habit of building for one generation only. Somehow we must recapture the old spirit.

It must be admitted though, that long-term responsibility can lead to awkward, and even tragic conflicts. I said in Chapter 3 that it is an ethical imperative to feed the starving, and to feed them well, even if it were proved beyond a shadow of doubt that a hundred years hence we shall run into a Malthusian limit. But it is equally imperative that those born a hundred years hence shall not starve! The conflict can only be solved by lacing the food with sterilizing agents, or by other means to the same effect. If this is rejected as 'interfering with sovereignty' or 'racial insult', there may be no solution.

As I have previously said several times, I consider it to be axiomatic that the mature society must maintain all the time the *maximum* of freedom which is compatible with social stability. How do we decide on such a question at present? It is fought out between pressure groups of radicals, liberals and conservatives. Each of these has a model in his mind, always incomplete, usually contradictory. In the best case one of the groups can point to experiences in another country; for instance, those who want to abolish every trace of censorship point to the repeal of the obscenity laws in Denmark. But conditions are never quite the same. The prohibition laws in Sweden caused little trouble, in the United States they led to the largest increase ever in organized crime.

Here again I see hope in computer simulation. We can put to the computer questions such as: 'What will happen if we legalize marijuana smoking? Is the number of hard drug addicts likely to increase or to decrease?' – 'What will happen if we abolish the death penalty, exempting (or not) the murder of police officers?' – 'What will happen to crime if we outlaw violence on television?' The last problem is a good example of the type which it is absolutely impossible to decide by orthodox empirical methods. One would have to take a sample of, say, 1000 American children, exposed to the daily violence on the screen, and a control sample of another 1000 whose parents would turn off the TV before every programme which contains violence. But those boys and girls who would submit to this without slipping to the house next door would be an exceptionally obedient sample, and the whole experiment would be worthless, quite apart from the fact that one would have to follow the fate of the children for at least twenty years.

But how can we obtain the quantified psychological data which have to be fed into the computer, such as the propensity to escapism or to crime, suggestibility, the influence of the environment? We certainly cannot do this today. We have not got the data, nor have we the army of trained psychologists who could supply them. We have many intuitively gifted psychologists among our enthusiastic educators, but they must first be trained in quantitative thinking. It will be also necessary to test if not all children, at least very great samples of them with very recondite test batteries, and to obtain an idea of the reliability of these tests by having every child tested by at least two psychologists. One cannot expect every problem to be 'well-conditioned', such as Forrester's town models, which were rather insensitive to the assumptions. In the case of 'ill-conditioned' problems, which show a wide spread of results depending on the data, the advice of the computer may be disregarded.

I do not think that one can raise very valid objections to such mass tests in the sacred name of privacy. We know that those who can afford it are keen to reveal their innermost life to psycho-analysts. And as regards the army of highly trained testers, I believe that social psychology will be one of the most rewarding intellectual professions of the near future.

19. MAN IN A MATURE SOCIETY

In our days nobody dares to paint a Utopia: a picture of a desirable, stable, more or less stationary world, towards which we must consciously strive. But meanwhile the idea of a stationary, stable ecosystem has come in through the back door, not by the work of imaginative writers, but by the sober estimates of econometricians, backed by computers, such as described in the last chapter. We have no choice other than gradual approach to a stable ecosystem or drifting into catastrophe.

In the previous chapters I have tried to follow a line which Karl Popper has called 'piecemeal social engineering', sketching various single features of the transition period in education, employment and economics. Now I cannot shirk answering the fundamental question of how these features will fit together in a consistent world, and how man will fit into it. What can we offer him? The first thing we must offer him is *hope*.

THE ENGINEERING OF HOPE

'Man cannot live without hope' has always been true, but hope meant very different things. For primitive man it meant the hope of a successful hunt and gorging himself with meat. We moderns, used to regular meals, can hardly imagine what an orgy it was when the bellies could be filled to bursting. Later on, in agricultural societies, hope was focused on a good harvest and their rain rituals give us some idea of its intensity. In the times of despair, which followed the decay of the antique civilizations, hope was deferred to a life in the hereafter. In modern times hope became identified with annual growth in wealth and material comfort.

Must we reconcile ourselves to the dismal thought that this hope is now nearing its end through the frustration which comes with fulfilment in a stationary society, however wealthy, in which growth will unavoidably come to a halt? I believe that such a tragic conclusion is unwarranted. Hope is an *individual* value, it was a great mistake of our industrial society to make it a *group-collective* value. It is still an individual value for the professional man, who has the hope of climbing the social ladder until his retirement. But the average manual worker, who earns standard wages from the age of 20 until his retirement, has no such hope, and the position of the small clerk is not very different. His only hope is that he will get his share of the annual growth of wealth, and that his trade union will secure his share, or a little more if possible. This has led to the modern form of class war, which I have discussed in several places. I have also said that we cannot entirely avoid it in a free society, in which a certain amount of fight has become a psychological necessity, but we can mitigate its worst effects by making it less of a 'free-for-all'. But the best way of mitigating it is by breaking the lifelong tie between a man and his class or occupation and by giving individual hope to everybody.

A chance for a change of occupation is an old idea in socialist and Utopian literature (it probably originated with Fourier). The young Marx has strangely distorted it in his often quoted dictum: 'In communist or socialist society, all professions would, as it were, become hobbies; there would be no painters, but only people who among other things spend their time also on painting; people, that is, who "do this today and that tomorrow", who hunt in the morning, go fishing in the afternoon, raise cattle in the evening, are critics after dinner, as they see fit, without for that matter becoming hunters, fishermen, shepherds or critics.'* 'Raising cattle in the evening' is manifestly absurd, and one wonders whether Marx has not for once shown a sense of

* Karl Marx, *Deutsche Ideologie*, 1844, quoted e.g. by Hannah Arendt, *The Human Condition*, Univ. of Chicago Press, 1958, p. 118.

humour. Such a life, fit for country gentlemen, does not show any sign of developing in the communist countries.

We may not be able to efface all boundaries between work and play, as Marx seems to have hoped, but we can ensure that no man or woman need be tied to the same repetitive job throughout life. I am aware that this is not a universal cure. Works engineers and foremen have often proposed a change of jobs, especially to girls, who to all appearances have become stale and bored to death, only to be met with a determined refusal. There is also the experience of psychiatrists, that repetitious handiwork is excellent occupational therapy. But these are manifestly pathological cases. It is not always easy to separate them from the norm, because every child wishes the same tale to be told every night with the same words, and much of the child can survive in some adults. I believe, though, that most healthy people will welcome a chance of changing their occupation at least once in life, especially when their early education has saved them from falling into mental inertia.

The old Japanese practice, of paying workers in the same job wages which increase with age, may be somewhat better than ours, because it contains an element of hope, but it is very much a second best to a change in occupation. It conflicts with social mobility, and it is now falling into disuse even in Japan.

I will not go into too much detail on the engineering of hope, because it is a very great subject, and although the principle is general, each case ought to be handled individually. I have already suggested that after some years of production work, all workers should have the chance to take up a service occupation which brings them into personal contact with people, and that it is urgently necessary to remove the stigma from personal service. Those gifted and willing ought to have a chance around the middle of life to take a hand at teaching, and be rewarded by the contact with young people. All ought to have sabbatical years, in which they can enjoy increasing their knowledge if they are capable of it, learn a new profession, or at least acquire hobbies for their old age. And all who have done their stint of work, must be able to look forward to a retirement free from material worries. Add to this the very justified expectation that medical

science will free old age of many of its infirmities, and I think
that there will be in the new world enough of that hope without
which man cannot live.

HOMO LUDENS

Johan Huizinga's classic of this title, written just before the
Second World War, has found very stern critics in our time. The
latest English edition (Temple Smith, 1970) carries a deprecatory
introduction by George Steiner, in which he writes: 'It is in the
best and worst sense a *jeu d'esprit*, the anecdotal discourse of an
erudite, somewhat crotchety amateur.' Pieter Geyl wrote:
'Being at heart a mandarin, an elitist steeped in the ideals and
comforts of high bourgeois culture, Huizinga takes a persistently
selective and nostalgic view of civilization.'

Whatever truth these quotations may reveal about Huizinga,
I think they reveal as much about the contemporary literary
elite, to which their authors undoubtedly belong. They do not
seem to have noticed how far we have already advanced into the
era of *homo ludens*, of Man at Play. Have they not seen how many
people open their newspapers at the sports page, or that in Britain
the most highly paid people are the popular entertainers, followed
only at a great distance by industrialists and bankers? Of course,
we do not play any longer at *masques* and pastoral scenes and we
do not dance around the maypole. Some of the grimness of the
19th century still persists, but the spirit of play has penetrated our
world perhaps as much as any other before it.

Play is not 'serious', though it can be played very seriously. It
is not 'real' life, the life of production, defence, material achievement, though it can absorb much of the diligence, courage,
ambition of the player, often more than he gives to 'real life'.
A game is an *artificial universe*; with milder rules, it does not
threaten with starvation, frustration or prison. It can be enjoyed
actively, or passively, vicariously as a spectator, with only a
fraction of the participation demanded by 'real', hard life.

Our contemporary literary men are so obsessed by the ugliness
of industrial civilization, so intent on showing it even more

meaningless than it is, so keen on deploring the human condition, that they are reluctant to admit that life for the masses is already much less hard than it used to be. Unless we run into catastrophes, it is bound to be even easier. I suspect that many of our modern writers have as much of a dislike for the vulgarity of a comfortable mass-civilization as has Huizinga, whose nostalgic elitism they so resolutely reject.

There are essentially three ways in which non-destructive man can be happy; by creativeness, personal contacts and play. There is no hard and fast division between these categories. Much playfulness can go into love, and some past civilizations have made elaborate games of it.* Nor is there a boundary between artistic creativeness and play. Huizinga's greater predecessor, Friedrich Schiller, has expressed this in his famous words:

'Man shall *only play* with beauty, and he shall play *only with beauty*.'†

The great idealist was somewhat carried away by his vision of classical Greece, which idealized its gods and goddesses as beautiful, playful rascals, and in its art represented them with smooth foreheads, unwrinkled by the serious thoughts of mortals. It would be going too far in optimism to imagine our descendants as happy children, with unwrinkled foreheads, with no worry more serious than moonshine, but I believe that we have already made a modest progress towards playfulness since the grim, puritan Victorian times.

The mere enumeration of the plays and games in our contemporary civilization would fill a page, but it must be admitted that there is not much grace and beauty in them. What there is of grace and beauty, as in opera and ballet, is the inheritance of aristocratic centuries. (Note with what devotion the Soviets cultivate these old arts.) In the non-communist countries the young people are desperately trying to create new forms, from discotheques to mass rallies, but these are too strongly tinged with

---

* Beautifully described in Huizinga's other book, *The Waning of the Middle Ages*, Arnold, London, 1924.

† 'Der Mensch soll mit der Schönheit *nur spielen* und er soll *nur mit der Schönheit* spielen.' Friedrich Schiller, *Uber die ästhetische Erziehung*, Schillers Werke, Nationalausgabe, Weimar, 1962, p. 359.

protest to be aesthetic successes. Perhaps when there is not so much to protest against, the young people may succeed in creating new forms with grace and beauty.

For a generation, or perhaps two, while we are going through the crisis created by crowding and the conflict between the old values and the new, there is little hope of a new harmony. In this transitional period, unless all the free time and energy liberated by the relaxation of economic scarcity is taken up by love and play, the destructive instincts of man will take over.

TOWARDS A PLURALISTIC SOCIETY

In the era of economic scarcity and almost incessant wars the first value was survival. This required rigid hierarchical structures, which tended to be more rigid and to survive longer than was justified by necessity. Ancient Sparta, so highly praised by Plato, is an example of a State which remained in a condition of artificial barbarism in the name of national survival. The feudal system, which subjected the agricultural population to abject serfdom, with the thin excuse that they were protected by the strong arm of the knights, is an even more telling example of a social fraud committed in the name of safety and survival.

In our time the rigidity of our social and economic system, which was created in the epoch of scarcity, is being increasingly questioned by many authors of whom perhaps Herbert Marcuse has been the most influential.* There is much in Marcuse's criticism that is sound, but his rather obscure writings have so little positive content that it is not surprising that he has been made, at least for a time, the prophet of anarchism by revolutionary

---

* From the Political Preface which Herbert Marcuse wrote in 1966 to his book which first appeared in 1955: '*Eros and Civilization*: the title expressed an optimistic, euphemistic, even positive thought, namely, that the achievements of advanced industrial society would enable men to reverse the direction of progress, to break the fatal union of productivity and destruction, liberty and repression – in other words to learn the gay science (*gaia sciencia*) of how to use the social wealth for shaping man's world in accordance with the Life Instincts in the concerted struggle against the purveyors of Death'. So far so good, but unfortunately what follows is almost wholly negative.

youth. First let us smash up the 'establishment'; we will think later of what to put in its place! Anarchy has never worked in the past, it will work even less in a crowded, unavoidably highly complicated civilization.

The pressure of necessity is relaxing under our eyes in the highly industrialized countries. Not so long ago there were only a few thousand in many millions who savagely refused the straitjacket of regular work – the tramps. George Orwell has given us a fascinating account of this strange race.* Today the voluntary gipsies, many of whom live in colonies, can be counted by the tens of thousands; they call themselves beatniks, hippies, etc. Are these savages the precursors of the free, leisured, *diversified* men and women of the future? One may be allowed to doubt this, because with their long-haired, unwashed appearance they are more uniform than the despised 'squares'. Yet we cannot dismiss the question so easily.

There are now more than 2000 'communes' in the United States, and at least 100 in Britain, whose members have tried to separate themselves from the mainstream of industrial civilization. They are mostly small, with 5 to 15 members, and their average life is three to five years. This is not a new phenomenon; in Britain such colonies have existed for at least 300 years.† In the past they originated either from dire economic necessity or from nonconformist religious beliefs, often from a mixture of the two. The life of the religious communes, such as the Hutterites or Mennonites (one could also mention the Mormons, though they have now spread far beyond their commune), appears to be unlimited. Another long-lived type, the kibbutzim in Israel, form a rare exception, because they are sustained by a strong national will rather than by nonconformism. The life of the communes founded by economic nonconformists always tended to be short. Small groups of workers and artisans fled the towns to work a piece of land together, manufacturing their simple necessities by hand and trading only the unavoidable minimum with outsiders. In a few years these communes were ended by economic

* George Orwell, *Down and Out in Paris and London*, London, 1933.

† W. H. G. Armytage, *Heavens Below*, Utopian Experiments in England 1560–1960, Routledge & Kegan Paul, London, 1961.

bankruptcy, but more often by internal quarrels. The colonists are not a random sample of the population, they are usually rather more intolerant and hard-headed than the rest, and those who are misfits in the mainstream of society very often find that they do not fit into a small commune either. At present dissension is probably even more often the cause of the breaking up of communes than before, because in a rich society even those who do not work enough or do not work at all can find it comparatively easy to live by begging or borrowing.

On the whole the story of nonconformist communes is a dismal one, yet I believe that a mature society ought not only to tolerate but to foster them. In the first place, they are a safety exit for rebels who would have a disruptive effect if they were left in the mainstream. A few years in a commune may cure them, but even if they spend all their life in communes, they will more or less sustain themselves economically, and will do less harm than if they form nuclei of disorder. A rich society does not need the work of all. There is, however, a more important reason why I would encourage rather than discourage nonconformism. Communes may well become the germ of that *diversity* without which the civilization of tomorrow might remain just as dull and monotonous as that of today.

Communes need not remain refuges for cranks, misfits and simple-lifers, let alone for sexual experimenters or junkies. They could well become sub-societies of creative individuals, who prefer to live in close union with other like-minded people. There would be no need for them to waste their time growing their own food; a rich society could provide them with the primary necessities. They could then build their own distinctive villages and towns, as small groups of monks in the past have built their own churches. Let these small towns compete with one another in originality, let them be as diverse as now they are uniform and dull. If their originality is not sufficient to create something new, they could fall back on old patterns. Modern man may have a nostalgia not only for more Williamsburgs and Rothenburgs-ob-der-Tauber, but also for medieval fishing villages, even for prehistoric lake-villages, not as museum show-pieces, but with their distinctive modes of living.

Nor need eccentric communes be technologically primitive. I can imagine that when the mainstream of civilization becomes life-oriented, there will be some archaically-minded people who will hanker after the old-fashioned ideas of technological progress, and play at making life-like robots. On condition, of course, that it remains a play, like the automata of the 17th century.

Nor need communes be territorially compact. I can imagine that when the nations have long given up spending taxpayers' money on the exploration of the barren planetary system, there will still be people who will be interested in it. They could then form an international club, and finance space flights, just as Jules Verne imagined that the Baltimore Artillery Club would finance the first flight around the moon.

All this would form a sort of pluralistic society, one in which individuals with nonconformist scales of value are not only free to have hobbies, but are free to ally themselves with like-minded people to realize their dreams. A rich society could afford it; what it cannot afford is boredom and frustration.

Hope, play, diversity; these are three offerings of a mature society to man, which perhaps may go some way to reconcile him with his fate: to be happy.

20. SUMMARY AND OUTLOOK

An ordered retreat is the most difficult of military operations. The transition from a society which idolizes growth to a mature one will be hard, because it means a retreat in many of the dimensions in which our world is now 'progressing'.

We are progressing towards an impossible growth of world population. Instead of unification, we have now some 140 'sovereign' nations, and even vigorous separatist, 'regionalist' and 'ethnic group' movements in some of the old-established great nations. The military technologies still keep developing apace, though we already have enough weapons to destroy the whole world population. The momentum of the established industries keeps producing more motor cars, more solid waste, more throwaway goods, more pollution. The population tends to concentrate in urban districts, in suburbias, while the centres of cities are decaying. In the non-communist countries the 'free-for-all' of labour and employers has created galloping inflation, which causes permanent economic unrest. All these are vigorous, self-sustaining tendencies, which will have to be stopped and reversed.

Our ideological preparation for dealing with these problems is very inadequate.* An important fraction of university youth has become very impatient, but their movements are conspicuously lacking in constructive ideas. There are many thinking people, politicians not excepted, who are longing for a vision, but

* For a fuller discussion of this, see Donald N. Michael, *The Unprepared Society*, Harper Colophon Books, New York, 1968.

168

are overwhelmed by day-to-day work* and by a feeling of impotence. Many feel that we are on collision courses, but do not know how to alter them. Stopping the machinery is not enough; any fool can do it, and there are enough fools busy doing it.

It appears that the widespread uneasiness has produced a healthy reaction in the new futurist movement. There is now a growing interest in the future, intensified by the approach of the millennial year 2000. A recent survey by the Council of Europe in Strasbourg list no less than 293 organizations in Europe which are interested in long-term planning and forecasting.† There are probably about as many in the United States.

The modern futurists are markedly distinct from their fore-bears: the political radicals, the Utopians and the technocrats. They are mostly politically uncommitted. They have among them a strong contingent of 'numerates', of people used to and skilled in quantitative thinking – econometricians, mathematicians, engineers. But they are not 'technocrats'; they do not have the naïve belief that all our world needs is better organization of production and more consumption.

All long-term social planning must start from two bases – the knowledge of Man, and the knowledge of material possibilities. It is understandable that quantitative futurist studies have so far been concerned with material possibilities, and that they have shied from taking their premises from that very obscure thing – the Nature of Man. This was justifiable so long as it was a matter of satisfying man's primary needs, but with the progress of technology and the expansion of possibilities which it brings with it, the psychological reactions to technological and cultural change become more important, and more threatening. At some future time the two lines of knowledge may merge into a new science, which I would call 'The New Anthropology'; the science of stable human civilizations at a high level of material comfort, but this may be several generations away. As the problems before

---

* The United States Congress has to deal with 10,000 bills annually. It is true that many of them are small ones.

† Of these 101 are governmental, 113 non-governmental and 66 university bodies.

us are far too urgent, one is forced to take an intuitive approach. This is what I have attempted in this book, however unsatisfactory it may be to build on such unknown ground, and I am very much aware of the danger of pitfalls. I will now briefly summarize my premisses and some of my conclusions:

Premisses. We must work towards a mature society, stable in numbers and in material production, in ecological equilibrium with the resources of the Earth. We must maintain the maximum amount of individual freedom which is compatible with social stability.

Conclusions and suggestions. Man does not appreciate what he gets free and can take for granted. A permissive society is possible only if it cultivates personal responsibility and if coercion is replaced by individual discipline.

For a long time work must remain the principal occupation of mankind, but work will mean less and less the production of material goods. Services must become more and more important. Personal service (*not* by a permanent *class* of servants) is necessary to make the world an agreeable place. Personal service must be freed from the stigma which adheres to it from the time when it was little better than slavery.

It can be expected that by the turn of the century, what now constitutes the 'public sector' and provides most of the social services, will have grown from one-half to about three-quarters of the whole economy. It will be increasingly difficult to maintain this with taxpayers' money, and there will be a strong temptation to make the whole economy centrally administered. I believe that whatever happens later, in the transition period we must make the best use of *true* private enterprise. Much of what is now paid out of taxpayers' money must be made to *pay* for individual enterprise, through the customer. It must *not pay* for individual enterprise to create sprawling suburbs, traffic bottlenecks, or to damage the environment.

The de-stabilizing institutions and practices of our free economy must be reformed. The capital market must be made less suitable for speculation, and more suitable for the solid investment of savings in public enterprises, which are now financed with taxpayers' money. Wage claims must be settled on a nation-wide basis, synchronously, instead of by successive single combats.

The education which makes the citizen fit for a mature society must start in the family. Everybody must receive an education in parenthood, to discourage those who are unworthy of it, or who are not emotionally mature enough to be good parents.

Education between the ages of six to eighteen cannot be wholly permissive. Membership of a rich, permissive society will not be appreciated without a hard apprenticeship. In these years the history of our hard-won civilization must be driven deep into the consciousness, as if the boy or girl had lived through it. They must be made *viscerally* conscious of their responsibility to society and to the ecosystem.

Higher education must be split into two branches. There should be universities of the traditional type for the gifted minority, to prepare them for intellectually exacting professions. For the less gifted majority the mass university should be the entrance into the permissive society. Its assignment will be less vocational training than giving them a taste for culture and life-long self improvement. It may teach them foreign languages, preparing them for years spent abroad, making them citizens of the world. The mass university must be an agreeable place, to which the students will be glad to return later in their sabbatical years.

Those capable of it must be given a chance to change their occupation in middle life. Nobody ought to be tied for life to a monotonous production job. Service occupations must be made rewarding by the opportunity for personal contacts, and by social esteem for those who are good at it. Almost everybody ought to take a turn at them.

Life must be made richer by not only tolerating nonconformists, but by actively encouraging those who can creatively add to its diversity.

Finally two short slogans, which would go a long way if they were obeyed:

Excellence instead of quantitative growth.
Possession instead of consumption.

The first is an advice to the industrial elite, the second to everybody. Possessions which do not wear out, not only material possessions such as beautiful habitations, but also arts, knowledge and the memory of a life rich in fulfilments.

Who can be the carriers of a programme like this? From beginning to end it is a list of *compromises*. Compromises between freedom and order, between human nature and social necessity. Such a programme cannot be made into a platform for a political party. It contains no encouragement for villain-hunting, which might make it attractive to young rebels. It is a Fabian programme, which aims at introducing reforms gradually, without hurting anybody. Nevertheless, it is certain to come up against strong opposition, because it conflicts with some modern shibboleths, especially by the advocacy of hardship in education, and by the explicit recognition of the inequality of men in the proposal to split higher education.

No such programme can be made into a banner for a mass movement, so I must confess again to unashamed elitism. Only an elite can carry it through, but this does not mean that I propose a society controlled by 'technocratic mandarins'. Such a movement need not conflict with democracy any more than did the movement of the Fabians, who were an elite of exceptional intellectuals.

The term 'democracy' has been discredited by the communist countries, which loudly claim to be democratic while denying the fundamental right in a democracy – the right of the people to make political choices. But many true democrats on our side have also regretfully recognized the limitations of this great political idea. For instance, Bertrand de Jouvenel has asked how we could put questions to the electorate such as this: 'How to maintain steady growth at $3 \cdot 5\%$ per annum, a positive balance of payments, less than 2% unemployment and steady prices?' It is clear that democracy must be reinterpreted.

I believe that a workable compromise has been created centuries ago in the ingenious invention of the *jury system*. Ordinary citizens on the jury listen to both sides, but in the end they bring in their verdict on the basis of instructions by a learned judge. In a liberal democracy we cannot prevent the citizen from being influenced by interested parties and by the slogans of extremists through the press and the mass media, but we may be able to educate him to pay serious attention to a detailed, impassionate exposition of the pros and cons by experts.* At present we have no social-political equivalent of the learned judge, but in the chapter on the art of prediction I have indicated that there is hope of such expertise becoming available in the future.

Normative programmes, such as I have sketched out, ought to be first discussed between my fellow-futurists and other experts, who could then elaborate those which they consider desirable and feasible into *projects*. They may then submit their plans (or preferably several alternative plans) for reaching agreed goals to governments, parliaments and public opinion. Once an idea has reached the project stage and is backed by adequate means, one can expect its success with a high degree of confidence. The art of coordination has magnificently developed in our times. We have seen how in the Apollo projects more than a half a million workers have collaborated in making many tens of thousands of parts fit together, and in bringing off the moon flights with split-second accuracy. I trust that if we could mobilize the right sort of intellects, they would collaborate with equally great enthusiasm in social projects. Once a start is made, I would expect such projects to spread over most industrialized countries. It is up to the United States to take the lead. They are the strongest, and also most in need of regaining their self-confidence which has been badly shaken by recent events.

Can a great new civilization arise from all this confusion around us, a civilization which can be compared with the great creative epochs of the past? I think that, even taking a very sober

---

* This may be made easier by the fact that most *really* important decisions cut right across party-political lines. This was the case in Britain with the abortion and homosexuality laws, the abolition of the death penalty and the question of entry into the Common Market. Incidentally, all were carried *against* a popular majority.

view, we cannot doubt that an educated population, conscious of its great cultural heritage, living mostly in small planned cities, designed by gifted architects, will develop a better artistic appreciation than those who are now living in the hideous small towns or neurotic big cities of Britain or the States. I cannot believe that they will accept imbecile 'happenings' and soup-tin collages as 'art'. With a great part of their energies freed from acquisitiveness and petty strife there may be even an awakening of human talents, which, in Lewis Mumford's words, 'may make the Renaissance look like a stillbirth'. And perhaps there will appear that lovely mutant, that joyful creator, 'Mozartian Man'.

Such lofty ideals, like happiness, cannot be approached in a straight line. Almost all the present trends of our world are against us: overpopulation, nationalism, economic group inertia and general aimlessness. Our best potential ally, youth, is deeply confused. All this must not discourage the truly creative intellects among us. If they rise to the real great challenge of our times, mankind may be able to step on a higher plateau without, as usual, first falling into an abyss.

POSTSCRIPT

In several places in this book I have pointed to Sweden as the democratic laboratory of the future. The Nobel Prize in Physics, which I received in December 1971, at last gave me an opportunity to collect some first-hand information. The quality of my informants made up for the shortness of time. Undoubtedly, a Nobel Prize winner is inclined to see Sweden through rose-tinted spectacles. But even allowing for this bias, I think that I was justified in deriving considerable encouragement from these interviews. The democratic Utopia, free enterprise under a very close state supervision, *works*, if not perfectly, at least as well as somebody with my strong misgivings about human nature can expect.

First the shadow side. An interview with Professors Delbom, Berglund and Holmer of the University of Uppsala confirmed my suspicions about the type of informal, permissive education which has been in force in Sweden since the early 1960s, and which has now spread into secondary education. Classroom chaos at the lower levels and truancy in high school are now so widespread that a parliamentary committee has been appointed to investigate. The standard of attainment has sunk to previously unrecorded depths. It remains to be seen how these youngsters will behave when they grow up. For the time being the situation is not too bad. The famous *raggare*, the moronic gangs whose fun it is to provoke the police and to be beaten up, really exist, but, as I heard from the Police Department of Stockholm, they number only about 2000, which is not too many for a city of over a million. Balance this against the other wing of youth, the students of the University of Stockholm: a finer and gayer body of young people I have never met.

Minister Moberg and Prime Minister Olaf Palme kindly granted me long interviews. In the past twenty-five years of socialist rule in Sweden their first object was to improve the housing of the working people. They can justly be proud of their achievement; it is estimated that half, perhaps even more, of the workers in Stockholm have a second home, outside the town. The Swedish achievement in retraining, already mentioned on p. 98, is also unique, and a model for the world. They are not unduly worried about unemployment, which has now reached about 100,000, mainly due to the drop in exports. Forecasts indicate that it will change into a roughly equal excess demand for workers in the next decade, without any large-scale redirection into service occupations, and still with the main emphasis on production.

Their main objective in the next twenty-five years will be the improvement of working conditions. A Government concentrating on *ergonomics* in a country like Sweden cannot fail to achieve spectacular results.

So let us look to Sweden as the vanguard of the free world. They are so far ahead of the rest of us, that we can learn from their mistakes as well as from their successes.

4 January 1972

NOTES

NOTE 1 (Chapter 1) *The Class War in Britain, 1951–69*

In Britain, between 1951 and 1969, retail prices increased by a factor of 2·0 and the average weekly earnings of manual workers by a factor of 3·2. Thus there was a real gain of 60% in 18 years, which is a little less than 2·5% per annum. The pay of salaried workers increased almost exactly in step.

Class warfare never ceased in these years, yet it made a surprisingly small impression on the distribution of incomes. The table below is taken from *Social Trends*, No. 1 (edited by Muriel Nissel, HMSO, London, 1970, p. 88).

COMPOSITION OF TOTAL PERSONAL INCOME IN THE UNITED KINGDOM

Source of income	1951	1961	1966	1967	1968	1969
Employment	71·3	71·7	70·9	70·2	69·9	70·5
Self-employment	12·0	9·2	8·3	8·4	8·1	7·6
Rent, dividend and net interest, etc.	10·6	11·6	12·0	11·9	11·8	11·6
National insurance benefits and other current grants from public authorities	6·0	7·5	8·8	9·5	10·2	10·2

It is clear that the 'working classes' have not been able to wrest any income from the rent- or dividend-enjoying 'capitalist class', who even increased their share slightly. In fact the employees have gained a little, because about 90% of the national insurance benefits go to employees and ex-employees, so their total share has increased from 76·8% to 79·7%. This, however, was at the expense of the self-employed, who include doctors, lawyers, etc., but also such 'small capitalists' as shopkeepers. This was all the benefit from 18 years of industrial disputes, intending to get a larger slice of the cake. One can of course contend that without this the *rentiers* would have increased their share even more. Perhaps we have been really living in the world of *Alice Through the Looking-Glass*, where one has to run very fast just in order to stand still.

There is not much that the lower brackets could gain, even with the most ruthless expropriation from the 'rich'. If *all* the after-tax incomes above £2000 per annum were taxed away and distributed among those with less than £2000, the latter would gain 14% – but of course the whole cake would collapse!

NOTE 2 (Chapter 1)

One may well wonder how much *paid* voluntary absenteeism is hidden in the astonishingly high figures for certified sickness in Britain, taken from Table 63 in *Social Trends*, Central Statistical Office, HMSO, 1970. The figures below were taken in 1967–68 on a 5% sample of the working population.

Days lost

Age	under 20	20–24	25–30	30–34	35–39
Male	6·6	7·1	8·0	9·3	10·7
Female	8·1	9·5	12·0	16·1	20·3

Age	40–44	45–49	50–54	55–59	60–64
Male	12·6	14·8	18·9	26·9	45·5
Female	22·5	27·3	34·9	44·6	—

The average for all ages was 16·4 days for males, 16·6 for females. The figure for females has remained practically constant since

1954, the figure for males had risen in the same period from 12·9 days to 16·4.

NOTE 3 (Chapter 1) *The Hawthorne Effect*

Everything works at first! This is widely known as 'The Hawthorne Effect'. Between 1926 and 1932 the Western Electric Company in their Hawthorne Works, Chicago, carried out a series of experiments in industrial psychology which have become justly famous. In one of these series a group of five girls, engaged in assembling of telephone relays, were put in a test room. First they were allowed to settle down, then they were tested under various conditions in 11 test periods of one to three months each. Their pay was made proportional to their output, the work period was shortened, rest pauses were introduced, refreshments given, etc. After almost every change there was a significant improvement in their output. In the twelfth period the original conditions were restored (without rest pauses, without refreshments, etc.) – and there was another significant increase in the output! These results seem to defy any correlation between output and working conditions; it is clear that work-satisfaction is not a static, but a history-dependent dynamic variable. But in the present case a simple conclusion can be drawn: almost any change worked, not so much because it was a change, but because the girls appreciated that somebody was seriously interested in their work.

The Hawthorne Experiment was first described by Elton Mayo, *The Human Problems of an Industrial Civilization*, 1933 (reprinted 1960 by the Viking Press). Later, in full detail, by F. J. Roethlisberger and W. J. Dickson, in *Management and the Worker*, Harvard University Press, Cambridge, Mass., 1939.

NOTE 4 (Chapter 4) *The Post-Industrial Society*

The term 'Post-industrial Society' has been coined by Daniel Bell (see for instance *Daedalus*, Summer 1967). His definition is considerably different from that of Herman Kahn. Bell considers it as the chief characteristic of the Post-industrial Society that its dominant figures will not be, as in the past 'the entrepreneur, the businessman and the industrial executive; the "new men" are the scientists, the mathematicians, the economists and sociologists, the practitioners of the new "intellectual technology" which is coming into being through the uses of the computer.' He forecasts an enormous increase in the number of professional and technical persons in the USA from 3·9 million in 1940 to 12·5 million by 1975, and an even steeper increase in the number of scientists (from 320,000 in 1960 to 650,000 in 1975) and of engineers (from 850,000 to 2 million, in the same period).

Daniel Bell may well be right in the short term, but in the long term I do not regard such a growth in numbers as either necessary or desirable. 'More means worse,' as Kingsley Amis has said, and if we increase the number, we produce just that type of second- or third-grade scientist or engineer who could be very well replaced by the computer. Beyond a certain number, they would constitute a Parkinsonian drag on the economy, because they will of course desperately resist being replaced by computers. I would rather approve of such an increase in people who have an *understanding* of science and technology, but find their place in administration and education.

Herman Kahn has taken the income level as the measure of industrialization, and his scale is as follows (H. Kahn and A. Wiener, *The Year 2000, A Framework for Speculation*, Macmillan, New York, 1967):

Five levels of per capita income and industrial development in the year 2000

1 Pre-industrial	$50–200
2 Partially industrialized	$200–600
3 Industrial	$600 to perhaps $1500
4 Mass consumption or Advanced Industrial	$1500 to about $4000
5 Post-industrial	$4000 to perhaps $20,000.

Beyond that stage comes the 'Post-economic Society'.

NOTE 5 (Chapter 4) *Joseph Schumpeter on the Future of Capitalism*
How long can we maintain capitalism, as the social form in which

individual enterprise has most successfully manifested itself in the past? I think that Joseph A. Schumpeter, in *Capitalism, Socialism and Democracy* (3rd ed., Harper Brothers, New York, 1950), has pronounced a valid verdict: 'Capitalism, then, is by nature a form or method of economic change and not only never is but never can be stationary. And this evolutionary character of the capitalist process is not merely due to the fact that economic life goes on in a social and natural environment which changes and by its change alters the data of economic action; this fact is important and these changes (wars, revolutions and so on) often condition industrial change, but they are not its prime movers. Nor is this evolutionary character due to a quasi-automatic increase in population and capital or to the vagaries of monetary systems of which exactly the same thing holds true. The fundamental impulse that sets and keeps the capitalist engine in motion comes from the new consumer goods, the new methods of production or transportation, the new markets, the new forms of industrial organization that capitalist enterprise creates.' (p. 82.)

'Faced by the increasing hostility of the environment and by the legislative, administrative and judicial practice born of that hostility, entrepreneurs and capitalists – in fact the whole stratum that accepts the bourgeois scheme of life – will eventually cease to function. Their standard aims are rapidly becoming unattainable, their efforts futile. The most glamorous of these bourgeois aims, the foundation of an industrial dynasty, has in most countries become unattainable already, and even more modest ones are so difficult to attain that they may cease to be thought worth the struggle as the permanence of these conditions is being increasingly realized.' (p. 156.)

Schumpeter's influential book is a closely argued demonstration of the ultimate doom of the capitalist system, but this did not make him a socialist.

NOTE 6 (Chapter 6)

Mansfield Parkyns, a Victorian eccentric, whose brilliant description of the Egyptian siesta, the 'kyef', I have quoted in *Inventing the Future*, spent three years in Abyssinia, 1847–50, which he

described in *Life in Abyssinia* (John Murray, London, 1953) – a
fascinating book (re-issued in 1966 by Frank Cass & Co., London).
His food was sometimes a half-burned piece of gazelle, sometimes
a handful of locusts, sometimes a 'good raw onion, which is not
a bad thing by way of luncheon'. But it appears that he enjoyed
rather than suffered hardship:

'As a general rule abstinence does no harm in these climates, but
on the contrary, it is always a good thing, and often necessary.
I never felt lighter in my life, or more free from the many ills
that vex humanity, than during this long period of semi-starvation.
Wounds of all kinds healed like magic, and I never knew what it
was to be lazy or fatigued. On one or two occasions I remember
being much astonished at the little I suffered from otherwise ugly
wounds about the feet. Once, in running down the stony and
almost precipitous path which leads to the Mareb, I struck my
bare foot against an edge of the rock, which was as sharp as a
razor, and a bit of flesh, with the whole of my left foot little toe,
was cut off, leaving only the roots of the nail. This latter I suppose
to have been the case, as it has grown all right again. I could not
stop longer than to polish off the bit which was hanging by a skin,
for we were in chase of a party of Barea... but was obliged to go on
running for about twenty miles that afternoon, the greater way
up to my ankles in burning sand. Whether this cured it I know
not, but I scarcely suffered at all from it the next day, and forgot it
the day after. Another day I was running after an antelope which
I had wounded, and in my eagerness jumped over a bush, and on
to the trunk of a fallen tree. Now it so happened that a bough
had once stood exactly where my foot now lighted, but, having
been broken off, had left a jagged stump, one splinter of which, of
about the thickness of a tenpenny nail, entering the ball of my
foot, passed so far through that the point appeared like a black
spot immediately under the skin, half an inch above the junction
of the third and fourth toes, towards the instep, and then broke
short off. I got my game, butchered it, and carried it home
(some two miles) with the splinter in my foot, which I then drew
out with a nail-wrench. A quantity of blood issued from the
wound, but, with the exception of a little stiffness for a day or two,
which however nowise prevented me from walking, I suffered

no pain at all. Now, had this occurred to me in Europe, and under a good European diet, I should have been at least a fortnight laid up with a bad foot.' (Vol. I, pp. 278–9.)

This agrees perfectly with the tales of the inmates of concentration camps, of stomach ulcers healed, etc., except that the prisoners did not even have the advantage of a hot climate. Shall we draw the conclusion that a good man, like a good dog, must always be hungry? One must add the cautionary note that the beneficial effects of semi-starvation were observed only in adults, with body and brains fully developed. Starvation in childhood and in the adolescent years prevents full development, not only of the body but also of the intelligence. Consequently starvation cannot be a part of the hardship in the years of education which I discuss in Chapter 13. It may well be a part, though, of posteducational adventures, such as Wells prescribed for the Samurai in his *Modern Utopia*, or of the 'Herculean Feats' of the elect in Yefremov's *Andromeda Nebula*.

NOTE 7 (Chapter 9) *The Mathematics of the IQ–EQ Diagram*

Let $x = IQ - 100$ and $y = EQ - 100$. A two-dimensional Gaussian distribution has the general law

$$\rho(x,y) = \frac{1}{2\pi} \frac{1}{\overline{x^2}\,\overline{y^2}(1-\rho^2)^{\frac{1}{2}}} \exp\left[-\frac{1}{2(1-\rho^2)} \left(\frac{x^2}{\overline{x^2}} + \frac{y^2}{\overline{y^2}} - \frac{2\rho xy}{(\overline{x^2}\,\overline{y^2})^{\frac{1}{2}}} \right) \right]$$

where $\overline{x^2}$ is the mean square dispersion of the IQ, and $\overline{y^2}$ of the EQ. I have assumed both to be equal to $\sigma^2 = (16 \cdot 14)^2$. (Or 16^2, or 15^2 according to newer definitions of the standard deviation.) ρ is the correlation coefficient

$$\rho = \frac{\overline{x \cdot y}}{(\overline{x^2}\,\overline{y^2})^{\frac{1}{2}}}$$

between the IQ and the EQ. If the distribution is Gaussian, the main interest of the problem is contained in this quantity.

The contour lines of equal probability density are ellipses

$$x^2 + y^2 - 2\rho xy = \text{const.} = R^2$$

with principal axes in the directions $\pm 45°$ and with a ratio of the long axis to the short axis of

$$(1+\rho)^{\frac{1}{2}}/(1-\rho)^{\frac{1}{2}}$$

The fraction of the population contained inside an ellipse R is

$$P = 1 - \exp[-R^2/2\sigma^2(1-\rho^2)]$$

In the diagram (Fig. 2) I have shown the contour lines for $\rho = 0$, zero correlation, in dotted lines, and for a reasonably strong correlation, $\rho = 0\cdot6$, in continuous lines. The axis ratio for these is $(1\cdot6/0\cdot4)^{\frac{1}{2}} = 2$. For equal values of $P - s$ (fraction of population inside R) the area of an ellipse is $(1-\rho)^{\frac{1}{2}} = 0\cdot8$ of the corresponding circle.

Though the IQs and the EQs have by our definition Gaussian distributions the joint distribution need not be Gaussian. The Gaussian distribution is distinguished by the property that the EQs for *any* IQ-bracket have a Gaussian distribution with the same standard deviation as the total, and vice versa.

NOTE 8 (Chapter 9) *Visualizing Multidimensional Distributions*
Recognizing characteristic 'shapes' in a multidimensional distribution is far from easy. The distinguished psycho-statistician Charles Spearman (a great critic of the IQ) has spent most of his life in trying to prove that the successes and failures of individuals in various examinations and tests are essentially determined by a single 'general ability factor', or 'psychophysical energy', without arriving at a convincing proof.

Imagine the results of various aptitude tests plotted on an N-dimensional space as coordinates. This gives a 'starry sky' in N dimensions. Are there correlations in it, has the whole cluster a narrow, elongated shape as Spearman has imagined, or are there perhaps distinct groups in it? If it were a two-dimensional distribution, a single glance would answer the question, in a three-dimensional distribution a few views from different angles. But when it comes to more than three dimensions, the methods of numerical analysis, even speeded up by modern computers, are very clumsy. For instance, if there is a suspicion that the distribution contains two fairly distinct groups, one must take a hyper-plane (an $N-1$ dimensional subspace), try all orientations and move it at right angles to itself in order to see whether there is a 'gap' which contains an abnormally low number of individuals. In two or three dimensions one could see this at a glance.

It may be useful to bring to the attention of psycho-statisticians that there exists an elegant electronic method which combines the power of computers with that of the human eye. Donald M. MacKay* has produced the electronic means for projecting three- (or more) dimensional structures on the face of a cathode ray tube and rotating those around any axis. (In N-dimensional space the rotation is around a hyperplane, which remains invariant.)

In order to apply this method to statistical distributions, the N coordinates (test results) of the individuals are stored, preferably digitally, in a magnetic tape or the like. These data are one after the other converted into analogues (coordinates) in rapid succession, and MacKay's rotational transformations are applied to them, by turning a number of knobs. There is no difficulty in transferring to the cathode ray screen 10,000 or even more bright points 50 times per second, so that the motion appears continuous. The observer tries out all orientations, but not blindly, because as soon as he perceives some degree of simplification, he can go on in the right direction until he arrives at an optimum.

NOTE 9 (Chapter 9)

The late A. H. Maslow, in his book *Motivation and Personality* (Harper & Row, New York, 1954), has an interesting chapter on 'Self-Actualizing People: a Study of Psychological Health'. Happiness is a characteristic of these fortunate people, but Maslow went a little too far, and my impression is that his personalities are nearer to 'supermen'. No wonder that among the 3000 students of Brandeis University he found only 3 fairly sure and

* D. M. MacKay, 'Projective Three-dimensional Displays', I and II, *Electronic Engineering*, July and August 1949, pp. 249 and 281. 'High Speed Electronic Analogue Computing Techniques', *JIEE*, 102, 609, 1955. Also *Multidimensional Displays* in London Thesis, 1950.

2 probable subjects, so that he had to eke it out by public and historical figures. Some of these were great creators, whose happiness I would characterize as 'proud and grim' (Spinoza, Beethoven and Freud among others). Nevertheless he found some characteristics, especially of the love relationships of such people, which may apply to ordinary men and women gifted for happiness (though singularly badly to Spinoza, Beethoven or Freud).

NOTE 10 (Chapter 13)

Sir Henry Churchill Maxwell Lyte, in his *A History of Eton College, 1440–1910*, writes of John Keate, 1773–1852, Headmaster of Eton between 1809 and 1834:

'Keate had no favourites, and flogged the son of a duke and the son of a grocer with perfect impartiality . . . he used to make point-blank charges of lying at random.' '. . . 1825, when on the 3rd February Keate is stated to have flogged forty-six boys in succession, for some offence unrecorded, and 80 on 30 June 1832.' (p. 269.)

'The masters were Anglican clergymen of the old type and the religion of the public school, if we can call it a religion, was crude in the extreme. The prevailing morality was the morality of the tribe, tyrannical, often barbarous. The bullying was severe, and the fags were often tortured by their fag-masters. As among the Spartan youth, certain forms of theft were accounted permissible, even honourable. . . . Rebellion against masters was frequent. Byron began his career as a rebel in the great Harrow mutiny which broke out in 1808 against an unpopular headmaster. . . . The first cricket match between Harrow and Eton was played in 1796, without permission of the respective authorities, and all the boys who took part in it were flogged.' (p. 468.)

NOTE 11 (Chapter 14)

Two years before C. P. Snow's Rede Lecture, Herbert J. Muller in his book *The Uses of the Past (Profiles of Former Societies)*, Mentor, London, 1957 (a book which in my opinion did not get the attention it deserved), wrote:

'The immense visions of modern physics and astronomy are considered less imaginative than the most tortured imaginings of modern poets, less spiritual than the mildewed metaphors of conventional churchmen. In general the limitations of modern culture are due not only to the narrowness of scientists and technicians, and the grossness of businessmen, but to the fastidious exclusiveness of literary and learned men, jealous of their traditional prerogatives as custodians of a higher and holier kind of truth.'

NOTE 12 (Chapter 14)

Three-dimensional projection with fisheye lenses realizes the same effect which the writers of SF and of fantasy stories expect from 'all-wall television'. This is nowhere near within the reach of technology (it requires an almost unimaginable waveband) which is just as well, because if it falls into the wrong hands, it might produce the effects which Ray Bradbury has brilliantly described in his *Fahrenheit 451* (1953). Guy Montag finds his wife Mildred reading her 'script', preparing for a TV programme in their parlour, with three walls rigged for TV:

'What's on this afternoon?' he asked tiredly.
She did not look up from the script again. 'Well, this is the play comes on the wall-to-wall circuit in ten minutes. They mailed me my part this morning. I sent in some boxtops. They write the script with one part missing. It's a new idea. The homemaker, that's me, is the missing part. When it comes time for the missing lines, they all look at me out of three walls and I say the lines. Here for instance the man says, "What do you think of this whole idea, Helen?" and he looks at me sitting center stage, see? And I say, I say – she paused and ran her finger under the line of the script, "I think that's fine!" And then they go on with the play until he says, "Do you agree with that, Helen?" and I say, "I sure do!" Isn't that fun, Guy?'

It takes a man with the fantasy of Ray Bradbury to reveal such a vision of the monumental inanity which the consumer society can produce.

NOTE 13 (Chapter 15)

J. L. Gray, a socialist, in a book on *The Nation's Intelligence* (Watts & Co., London, 1936), came to the conclusion that there may have been about as many talents in the 80% of the people who at that time had no access to university education as in the 20% who had. This agrees well with Lord Blackett's estimate.

NOTE 14 (Chapter 15)

Is history really cyclic? Herbert J. Muller wrote in his book *The Uses of the Past* (Mentor, London, 1957) on the medieval Italian universities: 'The only really strict rules were laid down by students to professors in the Italian universities, and enforced by threat of boycott. At Bologna the professors were compelled under oath to obey the Rector elected by the students, forbidden to leave the town for even a day without permission, fined if they began or ended their lectures a minute late, fined if they failed to attract an audience of at least five students for an ordinary lecture, and in general subjected to a very rigorous, but possibly salutary discipline. By the sixteenth century, however, the tables were turned; university regulation of student life was not only tightened but enforced. Thereafter students ceased to be gentlemen at large, and gradually turned into the schoolboys of today.'

NOTE 15 (Chapter 16)

In a meeting of the Bergedorfer Gesprächskreis (Discussion Circle Bergedorf-Hamburg, No. 32, January 1969) on the subject of 'Biology as a Technical World Power', Ernst von Weizsäcker remarked: 'Biological weapons could revolutionize not only warfare but also the technique of assassinations. For instance somebody could intrude into a parliament with a spray of certain bacteria. One can imagine the consequences. In all probability one could not even ascertain the assassin.' (We have come close to this when in 1970 a canister of CS gas was dropped in the British House of Commons, from the Strangers' Gallery, by a disaffected Irishman.)

Weizsäcker's conclusion is that not only wars must come to a stop, but also revolutions. Rebels ought to bear in mind that after a successful revolution the counter-revolutionaries will dispose of the same weapons. Unfortunately militants never seem to think of consequences beyond the first step.

When atomic weapons were invented, many of us congratulated ourselves that they were too complicated for madmen to produce them in their garrets or basement workshops. This, unfortunately, need not be true of biological weapons.

NOTE 16 (Chapter 16) *Dynamically Stable Suspension of Charged Particles in Oscillating Fields*

An electrically charged particle cannot be stably suspended in an electrostatic field, like Mohammed's coffin. There is nowhere a minimum of potential energy in which the particle could rest, as in a trough. It will unfailingly move towards one or the other of the electrodes, and join with an opposite charge.

In 1958 Ralph F. Wuerker and his associates H. Shelton and R. V. Langmuir* in the Ramo-Wooldridge Research Laboratories, Los Angeles, found a remarkable method of stabilizing charged particles, not statically, but dynamically, by alternating fields. The particle never comes to rest, but oscillates in orbits, closed or almost closed, and which can come very close to a central position, but never quite reach it. The precursor of this was the 'strong focusing principle', discovered in 1952 by Courant, Livingstone and Snyder, and the high-frequency electric mass filter of W. Paul and M. Raether.† In these devices a particle proceeds in a sequence of fields which are alternatingly focusing and defocusing, but if the alternation frequency is properly adjusted to the charge-to-mass ratio of the particle, the focusing will always prevail over the defocusing.

In the first of Wuerker's devices a charged dust particle is dropped into the space between two opposite, rounded electrodes, and a third, toroidal electrode, which forms a ring in the plane

* R. F. Wuerker, H. Shelton and R. V. Langmuir, *Journal of Applied Physics*, Vol. 30, pp. 342-9, March 1959.

† W. Paul and M. Raether, *Zeitschrift für Physik*, Vol. 140, pp. 262-73, 1955.

midway between the two. The two opposite electrodes are connected with one another. Whatever static voltages one applies between these and the ring, the particle will move towards an electrode with a charge opposite to its own. But apply on top of the static voltage an alternating voltage of sufficient strength and sufficiently high frequency, and the particle will be confined to a finite orbit. There exists a minimum frequency for stabilization. For small charged aluminium dust this is of the order of 50 cycles. The mathematical and experimental investigation shows that the particle executes a slow, large-amplitude oscillation around a central point, which one can easily follow with the eye, and a rapid oscillation, with the drive frequency, with small amplitude. The stability arises from the fact that during a 'microcycle' the force driving the particle backwards always prevails over that which drives it outwards. With a given frequency the device will accept all particles below a certain charge-to-mass ratio when the DC voltage is zero, while with DC present the acceptance can be made quite narrow.

NOTE 17 (Chapter 16)

Tying the claims of the unions together is by no means a new suggestion. William H. Beveridge advocated it very strongly in his great book, *Full Employment in a Free Society* (George Allen & Unwin Ltd, London, 1944) in which he proposed (i) stable prices, (ii) unified wage policy agreed by the Trades Unions General Council, and (iii) arbitration clauses in wage agreements. He wrote also with remarkable foresight: 'So long as freedom of collective bargaining is maintained, the primary responsibility of preventing a full employment policy from coming to grief in a vicious spiral of wages and prices will rest on those who conduct the bargaining on behalf of labour. But both the State and the managers of business have their parts to play. The part of the State lies in the adoption of a definite policy of stable prices . . . it is unreasonable to expect from trade unions a reasonable price policy, just as it is impossible to have a price policy without a wage policy.' (pp. 200-1.)

One may get some idea of the obstacles in the way of a unified wage policy from the fact that in Britain in 1968, there were 534 unions, all with a claim to independent bargaining. Shall we take hope from the fact that in 1951 there were 735 of them?

NOTE 18 (Chapter 17) *Statistical Freedom*

The theory of statistical freedom starts from the axiom that when choices are offered to a population, the freedom must manifest itself in a *spread* over the choices. But a spread is interpreted as a sign of real freedom only if it was not predetermined by conditions, called *factors*, which are not subject to choice, and which are undesirable *and* avoidable.

The freedom in choice of a profession may be again mentioned as an illustration. By the tenets of our democratic civilization we consider the social status of the father as an undesirable factor in the choice of the profession of the son. This is an avoidable influence in a society with free schooling and an anti-nepotistic climate of opinion. On the other hand we do not consider the IQ of the son as an undesirable factor, though one's IQ is just as little a matter of choice as one's father. There is no difficulty in sorting out desirable and undesirable influences in any civilization, though these may vary from one civilization to another.

The two basic features of freedom in a statistical theory are therefore *diversity* and *independence*. How can these be combined in one mathematical measure?

The raw material of any such measure are the choices made by the individuals in a population. For simplicity, let the choices be discrete, labelled by integer numbers i. These can be single choices, in which case i is one number, or multiple choices, in which case i is shorthand for a group of numbers (a vector in the 'i-space'). Similarly we label the factors (such as the social status of the father, or the income bracket) by numbers j, which can be also single or multiple. We then start from the fractions $p(i,j)$ of the population, which has made the choice i in the factor-group j. These fractions (which add up to unity) we call *preferences*. From these we want to construct an acceptable measure of freedom. Such a measure ought to satisfy the following six postulates:

1 If the whole population has made the same choice, its actual freedom was *nil*.

2 The freedom is also *nil* when there is diversity in the choices, but this is entirely determined by factors not subject to choice.

3 In all other cases the measure of freedom is a positive number.

4 The measure must never increase when new factors are taken into consideration.

5 The measure must never increase by finer subdivision of the factors.

6 The measure must never decrease by finer subdivision of the choices.

Postulates 1–3 are self-evident; 4 and 5 are conclusions from the principle of causality. Additional knowledge can never increase uncertainty. By postulate 6 an increase in recognized diversity must never decrease the measure of freedom.

André Gabor and I have shown in a first paper★ that there is an infinite variety of measures which satisfy these first six postulates, though we have singled out one of these for detailed discussion. In finding such measures we have used a heuristic method which in itself is of some interest. We have assumed that the distribution $p(i,j)$ of the preferences has come about by the population trying to make an optimum compromise between utility and freedom. We started from a 'social potential' Φ, which is the sum of a 'total utility' U and a 'total freedom' F. The choices i have certain utilities U_i, and U is the sum total acquired by the population. If the population were entirely homogeneous, and without any tendency to express individuality, it would concentrate on one choice, the one with the greatest utility. But because they are, to some extent, 'free', they will try to spread their choices, and this is accounted for by F, which is an 'entropy-like' function of the preferences, increasing with spread. The social potential Φ is therefore a close analogue of the thermodynamic potentials, such as 'free energy' which regulate the equilibrium of statistical systems in physics. From any such

★ D. Gabor and A. Gabor, 'An Essay on the Mathematical Theory of Freedom', *Journal of the Royal Statistical Society*, A **117**, pp. 31–72, 1954.

model one can derive a 'freedom coefficient', f_{ij}, by dividing the total freedom F which has been realized, by the freedom calculated by *ignoring* the conditioning factors. By this we satisfy postulates 4 and 5 because a conditional maximum can never be larger than an unconditional maximum.

The model has served well in deriving f_{ij} as a measure of freedom, but now it can be discarded, because the result speaks for itself. The freedom coefficient appears as the product of two factors, the *diversity* D_i in the choices i, and its *independence* I_{ij} from the factors j

$$f_{ij} = D_i I_{ij} \tag{1}$$

The first factor is a measure of the spread over the choices, i.e. of the diversity, and can be expressed in units of binary choices or 'duals'. The second factor is unity when the choices i are independent of the factors j and it is zero when they are completely determined by the factors.

There is a wide choice in 'entropy-like' functions F, and this leads to an arbitrariness in f_{ij} which it would be desirable to eliminate. We have shown in a second paper★ that one arrives at a *unique* measure by adding a seventh postulate:

7 The measure of freedom of a population is an additive linear function of the freedom of the groups of which it is composed, weighted with the numbers of the individuals in the groups.

This is the same axiom by which Claude E. Shannon arrived at a unique measure of information in his mathematical theory of communication.† The new, unique measure of freedom is

$$f_{ij} = - \sum_i \sum_j p(ij) \log p_j(i) \tag{2}$$

The notations are here the same as in Shannon's theory of com-

★ D. Gabor and A. Gabor, 'L'Entropie comme mesure de la liberté sociale et economique', *Cahiers de l'Institut de Science Economique Applique*, No. 72, pp. 13–25, Paris, November 1958.

† Claude E. Shannon and Warren Weaver, *The Mathematical Theory of Communications*, University of Illinois Press, Urbana, 1949, There exists now a vast literature on this subject.

munication, where the p stands for probabilities. $p_j(i)$ is the *conditional preference*

$$p_j(i) = p(i, j)/p(j) \qquad (3)$$

the fraction of individuals in the factor-group j who have elected the choice i. ($p(j)$ is the fraction of the population in the factor-group j, hence $p(j)$ is not a preference; p can here be interpreted as a 'population'.

The mathematical expression in equation (2) is identical with Shannon's 'conditional entropy'. The entropy in physics is, because of its additivity, a unique measure of the spread of a statistical system, or, in other words, of the uncertainty of its configuration. In communication theory the entropy is the measure of the uncertainty in an ensemble of messages. The informative value of a message is the reduction of the uncertainty which existed before the message was received. It may be noted that statistical communication theory has nothing to say about the semantic value of a message. Any 'yes' has the same value, whether it means the outbreak of a war, or just the next binary digit in a telephone number. The statistical theory of social freedom has the same feature. We do not propose 'exchange values', say, between the freedom to vote for one's party and the freedom to select a certain brand in a department store. We can compare like only with like, for instance the freedom in choosing a profession in different countries.

If in equation (2) we ignore the factors j we arrive at the unconditional entropy or diversity D_i:

$$D_i = - \sum_i p(i) \log p(i) \qquad (p(i) = \sum_j p(ij)) \qquad (4)$$

which is never less than the conditional entropy. From these we form, as in equation (1), the factor of independence $I_{ij} = f_{ij}/D_i$.

The factor of independence is a valuable tool for detecting and quantifying social constraints which may be desirable or undesirable. It is particularly useful for clarifying the influence of the factors and of their interactions if there are several lines of factors present. Unfortunately statistical tables with more than two entries are rare. We have been able to find only one trivariate table of considerable interest, the data on social mobility in Sweden, already mentioned in the text.* This lists the social class of fathers and sons (three groups each) and the IQ of the sons (eight brackets). This may be again used as an illustration.

The independence factor of the social class of the sons from the social class of the fathers is found to be 0·848; the independence from their IQ is 0·782. If both the social class of the fathers and the IQ of the sons is taken into account, there remains an independence from both factors of 0·705. It is more instructive to consider the 'factors of dependence' which are 0·152, 0·218 and 0·295. These have the interesting property that they are additive when the two factors are independent of one another. But in the present case they are far from independent, because the intelligence of the sons is not independent of the social class of the fathers. It would therefore be misleading to consider the influence of the social class of the father as only a little less than that of the IQ of the son. The *net* influence of the status of the father is obtained by deducting from the total dependence the influence of the IQ of the son, and this gives only 0·295 – 0·218 = 0·077. This suggests that social mobility in Sweden is not far from ideal. A more accurate judgment could be obtained only by comparing Sweden with other countries.

It would be most interesting to apply this method also to the often discussed question whether an ascent in the social scale gives more freedom or not. It has been suggested, especially in the United States, that it makes the individual even more hidebound, by forcing him to live in a certain type of house, buying certain cars, obliging him to send his children to expensive schools, etc. Adequate statistical material is not yet readily available.

NOTE 19 (Chapter 18) *The First World Model of the Club of Rome*
The systems diagram of the 'world-model' constructed by Professor Jay W. Forrester is too complicated, and has too much

* Gunnar Boalt and Carl-Gunnar Janson, *Social Mobility in Stockholm*, Congrès de l'Association Internationale des Sociologues à Liège, 1953.

detail, to be accommodated in the format of this book. A verbal description may be sufficient to understand its essentials. The system is built around five dynamic variants, called 'Levels':

> Population
> Natural Resources
> Capital Investment
> Fraction of Capital devoted to Agriculture
> Pollution.

The term 'level' is appropriate for these variables, because they are cumulative quantities, each with an outflow and an inflow, except the natural resources. These last are only the irreplaceables, such as oil or coal, which are steadily depleted. If substitutes are found, they must come *via* capital investments.

Once a level is given at a certain date, its future behaviour is determined by inflow and outflow. For instance the population increases by births, and decreases by deaths. Each of these rates has a 'normal' which has been adjusted so as to account for the global history of the level in question between 1900 and 1970. For instance the birth rate normal for the whole globe was 0·040 per annum and the death rate normal 0·028, giving for this historic period the slow increase rate of 0·012. According to the latest FAO reports this is expected to be about 0·021 for the next 30 years.

When the initial values of the levels and the rates are determined, the computer model can start making forecasts. If the rates were to remain constant, one would obtain naïve exponential extrapolations. The great merit of Forrester's model is that it makes an attempt at representing the very complicated inter-relations between all the levels and all the rates.

As in his previous industrial and city models, Forrester has dealt with these interrelations in a simple and ingenious way, by 'multipliers'. Consider the birth rate as an example. This is positively influenced by the availability of food and by the material standard of living (goods other than food), negatively by crowding and by pollution. The death rate is directly influenced by the same factors. Forrester replaces these influences by multipliers, each acting independently of the others. The 1970 values of the factors are considered as unity, and at these levels all multipliers are unity. If the factors depart from the standard value, the multipliers must be intelligently guessed. As an example

Material standard of living	0	0·5	1	2	3	4	5
Death rate multiplier	3	1·8	1	0·7	0·52	0·5	0·5

This is a reasonable guess, at any rate at high standards of living, because we know that in the highly industrialized countries a death rate (over long periods) of 0·014 has been achieved, corresponding to an average life of 71·5 years, and this is half the average of 0·028 over all countries, in the period 1900–70. As a second example:

Pollution level	0	1	10	20	30	40	50	60
Death rate multiplier	0·9	1	1·4	2·0	3·2	4·8	6·4	9·2

This appears somewhat more questionable, because we do not know with anything like sufficient precision the toxicity of pollution as a function of industrial activity. Opinions differ widely, and some would consider Forrester's death multipliers to be too pessimistic. But if it were true, as has been seriously suggested, that we are poisoning the phytoplankton in the southern seas, which digest 70% of the CO_2 in the air (far more than the green vegetation), Forrester's estimates might be on the optimistic side.

Forrester makes two assumptions. One is that all multipliers acting on one rate must be multiplied, the other is that each multiplier depends only on its own source. In brief, influences are *logarithmically additive*. This is a reasonable first approximation, and without it Forrester would never have been able to construct his models. Any further refinement will require an immense amount of statistical material, which is not available.

One can also object, that for instance birth rates are influenced not only by material levels, but also by religions, climates of opinion and legislation. (For instance, free abortion.) Such influences can be accounted for only by *interventions* in the model, corresponding to changes in policy, and this has in fact been done, as will be shown later.

There are fourteen such multipliers in Forrester's model, all quantitatively specified in his *World Dynamics*. These are connected with one another and with the rates by altogether sixty lines of influence, and these lines form a very great number of feedback loops, some positive, others negative.

The computer as described is an autonomous dynamical system, which once set in motion will trace out its future, taking a few minutes for a run covering a hundred years. Three such computer runs (a selection from a very great number), are shown in Figures 3 to 5. These graphs contain only four of the five levels, the capital investment in agriculture has been left out, but an important variate is added – the 'Quality of Life'.

The Quality of Life is not a dynamical variable, because it does not react on the system; it is an *indicator*, like a Social Welfare Function. This, too, Forrester has defined by four multipliers, two of which (Food Ratio and Material Standard) are favourable, two others (Pollution and Crowding) unfavourable. For any combination of these take the two data from the tables below, and multiply them.

FAVOURABLE FACTORS   Food ratio →

		0	0·5	1	2	3	4
	0	0	0·1	0·2	0·3	0·48	0·54
	0·5	0	0·3	0·6	1·05	1·44	1·62
Material standard ratio ↓	1	0	0·5	1	1·75	2·40	2·70
	2	0	0·85	1·7	2·96	4·10	4·60
	3	0	1·15	2·3	4·00	5·50	6·20
	4	0	1·35	2·7	4·70	6·50	7·30
	5	0	1·45	2·9	5·10	7·00	7·50

UNFAVOURABLE FACTORS   Pollution ratio →

Crowding ratio ↓	0	1	10	20	30	40	50	60
0	2·10	2	1·70	1·20	0·600	0·300	0·100	0·050
0·5	1·33	1·30	1·10	0·78	0·390	0·200	0·065	0·032
1	1·05	1	0·85	0·60	0·300	0·150	0·050	0·025
2	0·62	0·60	0·51	0·36	0·180	0·090	0·030	0·015
3	0·36	0·35	0·30	0·21	0·105	0·052	0·018	0·009
4	0·26	0·25	0·21	0·15	0·075	0·037	0·012	0·006
5	0·20	0·20	0·17	0·12	0·060	0·030	0·010	0·005

At present it is a matter of opinion whether one regards this as a reasonable measure of the Quality of Life. Later on one can perhaps establish by surveys whether the population is willing, for example, to put up with a crowding ratio of 2 in exchange for a rise in material standards by a factor of 5.

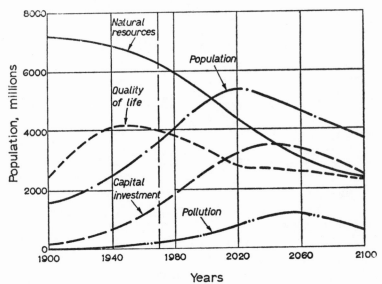

FIGURE 3   *First computer run. No change of policy in 1970. The quality of life is allowed to decline gradually.*

Figures 3 to 5 show the effect of three different policies on the fate of the world system to the year AD 2100. In all three the runs follow actual history between 1900 and 1970. The year of decision is 1970.

Figure 3 shows *no change in policy*. The quality of life, which has gently peaked around 1960, is allowed to decline slowly by exhaustion of natural resources. The population goes to a maximum of about 5300 million in 2020 and then declines slowly. (Note that this is well below the figure of 6500 million forecast by FAO for AD 2000.) Pollution also increases rather slowly, and this allows the quality of life to follow gradually a less steep decline. It reaches in 2100 about the same level as it had in 1900.

But we are not likely to put up with a decline in the quality of life. In Figure 4, in 1970, a decision has been taken to counter this

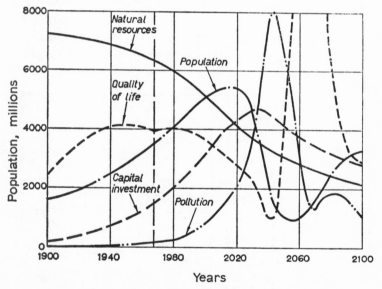

FIGURE 4 *In 1970 the rate of capital investment is increased by 20%*
in an effort to reverse the incipient decline in the quality of life.
Catastrophic consequences around 2030.

with a 20% increase of capital investment and thus a faster exhaustion of natural resources. This works for a while, but then it leads to catastrophic consequences. Around AD 2020 pollution shoots up so steeply that there is a drop in world population, without a parallel in history, to about one-fifth in 20 years. After this the quality of life shoots up. This is not quite without a parallel in history. Trevelyan records that the happiest epoch of medieval England was the half century which followed the great plague in the middle of the 14th century. After this the play seems to repeat itself.

All the policies which one would instinctively adopt for raising the quality of life leads to catastrophes in the long run. Those which lead to stable ecosystems appear highly unpalatable. One of these 'happy' runs is shown in Figure 5. Capital investment is reduced by 40%, birth rate cut to one half, pollution generation is reduced to one half of the 1970 level, the rate of the usage of natural resources to one quarter, and – most painful of all – food

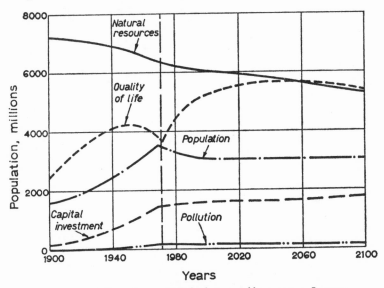

FIGURE 5 *A 'happy' run which leads to a stable ecosystem. In 1970 capital investment is reduced 40%, birthrate 50%, pollution generation 50%, natural resource usage rate 75%, and food by 20%.*

production is reduced by one-fifth. This policy would allow a world population of about 3000 million to survive, somewhat less than the present one, but at a much higher quality of life.

How seriously should we take such forecasts? I would say, very seriously as warnings to mend our ways, and to investigate ways and means for devising policies less cruel for avoiding eco-catastrophes. When the futurist ventures to make a prediction, it never means 'it will be so'. It always means 'it will be so if . . .' We always hope that sinister prophesies will be self-annulling. We also hope that benign forecasts will be self-fulfilling, but it must be admitted that the best-informed prophesies at present are the least optimistic.

I am very thankful to Professor Jay W. Forrester for letting me have in advance the manuscript of his *World Dynamics* from which I have abstracted this note.

INDEX